Carbon & Dust

2019

N. Rey | darebee.com

First Printing, 2019.
ISBN 13: 978-1-84481-018-5
ISBN 10: 1-84481-018-6

Warning and Disclaimer
Although every precaution has been taken to verify the accuracy of the information contained herein, the author and publisher assume no responsibility for any errors or omissions. No liability is assumed for damage or injury that may result from the use of information contained within.

Fitness is a journey, not a destination.
Darebee Project

Introduction

Carbon & Dust is an action-adventure with you as the main protagonist set in a distant future when humanity has spread far and wide across the Galaxy. It's a world where the corporations set and keep the laws and where you can only rely on your own strength, speed and cunning. To survive, you must become a weapon. To make a difference, you must be prepared to give it your all.

Enter the world of Carbon and Dust and see how far it'll take you.

This program can be completed one chapter per day (recommended). There is no preview to avoid spoilers. The program reads like a book with integrated action and tasks you must complete to advance further in the story.

Instructions

Reps (repetitions) per exercise are located next to each exercise's name. Number of reps is always a total number for both legs / arms / sides. It's easier to count this way: e.g. if it says 20 climbers, it means that both legs are already counted in - it is 10 reps each leg.

Before you start: Look over the workout you chose to do and make sure you understand all of the exercises illustrated so it doesn't slow you down once you have started.

Video Exercise Library darebee.com/video

Exercise Alternatives

If you are recovering from an injury, have a mild disability that prevents you from doing certain moves, have bad knees or are suffering from back pain and you want to avoid high impact exercises but you still want to stay active and try some of the workouts from this book, try these modifications.

The modifications will also be suitable if you are trying to keep the noise you make to a minimum.

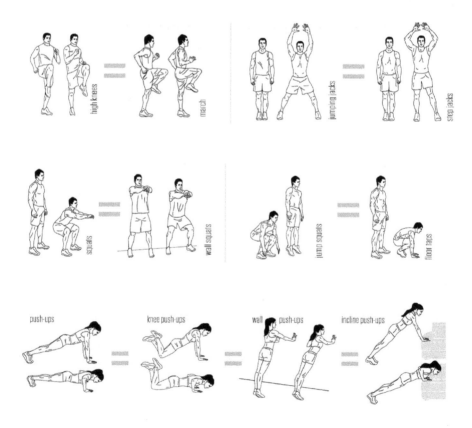

Chapter 1

It wasn't as painful as I expected. In fact, it ended with a quick "Zap" and an almost pleasant sensation of burning at the back of my neck. And just like that, all the weight of my past was gone. At some considerable cost of course.

It takes a moment to reorient. The brain has this thing: it requires memories to form an identity. That identity is partly formed by the biometrics stored in its hippocampus. I have kinda just changed mine. I say kinda because it's a veneer. It gets complicated so maybe I will explain it a little later on.

"All the biometrics are still the same but it won't flag it up," the tech is an older woman with a raspy voice. Bony with a full head of grey hair streaked with purple highlights. She runs through the code one more time. She raises an eyebrow in appreciation, admiring her work. "This is good work. As far as second chances go this is as good as it gets. I wouldn't stick around here for long however."

She is right. The whole point of a new bio ID is the option to start over, be someone else - somewhere else. I thank her, grab my gear and bolt. I have to be careful and fly under the radar until I get off this rock. There are still people here who don't need a bio reader to recognize exactly who I am. I am keen to avoid such encounters.

The moment I am out of the workshop, I throw my bag over my shoulder and start to run. It'll be safer if I made it across the station on foot, I don't want my new ID to register anywhere just yet, but I'd better hurry - the last ship leaving the planet until the end of the solar year will be gone in just a few hours.

It's still dark outside, I've timed it just right. The lights won't come on for at least the next two hours. Extra cover for me.

Makes it hard for the street cameras to capture my image.
I better hurry, though, I am cutting it close. There is the
familiar tightness of adrenaline in my system. I smile ferally
to myself. This one last time. Almost there, I say. Almost
there. I start to run.

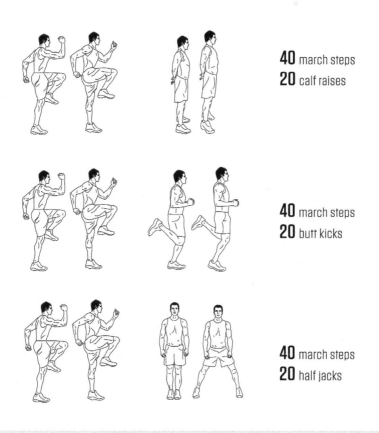

40 march steps
20 calf raises

40 march steps
20 butt kicks

40 march steps
20 half jacks

catch your breath, rest up to 2 minutes, and repeat the circuit
7 times in total

Suddenly I feel droplets of water landing on my face. Soon, small puddles start forming here and there. I could never understand why we have always brought our malfunctioning weather simulators to every planet regardless of its designation but there must be a good reason for this added misery. It was originally designed to help us adjust to the new environment and adapt so our psyche could handle it better but eventually it just became part of the standard package and no one has ever bothered to question it.

I heard you could never predict rain on our origin planet and here we are, still not being able to even schedule one when we have all the tools. It still catches everyone by surprise. Maybe it's a design flaw or maybe it's just part of the experience, something to do with being human.

I sigh. Now I have to mind the puddles, too. The weather however works to my advantage. It clears the streets of the few hangers-on and gives me a clear run to the station. It also means that there are fewer eyes around to see me which suits me just fine.

I take a shortcut skirting the main street. I pull my hood on and pick up the pace. Out of the corner of my eye I notice a holoposter, silver edge glinting at me as I pass through the rain.

RED REAPER REWARD
FOR INFORMATION LEADING TO THE APPREHENSION
OR DEATH ...

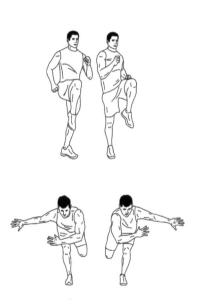

40 high knees

one jump to the left

40 high knees

one jump to the right

40 high knees

one jump to the left

40 high knees

one jump to the right

40 high knees

one jump to the left

40 high knees

one jump to the right

The rest of the beamed message is lost to me as my feet take me out of range.

Chapter 2

GT-701 planet is a mining colony. There is absolutely nothing special or even remotely interesting about it. GT-type planets are like that - they are a resource, once it dries out it's discarded and abandoned so we can move on to the next promising rock. No one makes places like this their home, not unless they have no other choice.

To me it has been a good place. I managed to do a lot here. Got my head straight at last.

Still, I will not miss it.

A pretty holographic face pops up from nowhere as I round a corner, probably a motion sensor picking me up. It's an ad:

"New Eden - The Paradise, Rediscovered! The highest standards of living on the most luxurious planet in the Galaxy! New Eden - you deserve it!".

I wave it away so it stops blocking my path. The ads are annoying but GT-type planets have no consumer protection legislature. There are even cases where a malfunctioning hoload has created such persistence planning that it's led to the psychotic breakdown of its unfortunate targets.
Talk about marketing gone wrong.

I am almost at the center of the station now, breathing hard. It envelops this side of the planet spreading in every direction like a spider-web with the operation center at the heart. It's a classic mining setup with all roads leading to the docks. It's the only way in and out of the planet, all operations start and end here.

My guess is from space it must look like a tick. It's there to suck the planet dry and when this planet has nothing to offer, the tick and everything that comes with it will disappear. Gone to suck some other planet dry. It's not a heartening thought and it annoys me. I should be feeling happier now. I am almost where I need to be, secure and happy. I just need to make this flight.

The main entrance is just ahead. It looks like I made it just
in time. I spot the skinny man with the precision goggles and
the dock uniform, he is the one I spoke to remotely. He is
supervising last minute loading of the shipment containers.
I wait until there is no one else around so I can talk to him.
I walk up.

"I am the off-manifest guest."
He looks around and quickly responds:

"I don't think so. No rats on board this time around."

"We had an arrangement..."

"Security is too tight, some important cargo or whatever. The
manifest is encrypted so there is nothing I can do. You can
either wait for the next round or we could work something
else out... but no cabin."

I can feel the storm rising inside but I quickly calm myself
down and dump down the emotion. Now's not the time to
lose it. I actually have too much to lose for once. I see what
he is doing: he knows this is the last ship off the planet for
a long time and he is gambling I'll be desperate enough to
pay more for less. If anyone is a rat here it isn't me. But he's
right. I am desperate to get away.

"How much?"

"I told you - the manifest..."

"Just tell me what do I need to do to get on that ship, today."

"Well, there might be a way..."

There always is.

"The chief of security has been on my ass with this shipment and really it would make my life so much easier if he missed this flight altogether. How it happens is up to you but if he isn't on board then I'll see to it that you are. He is not here yet so he must still be in the barracks, top floor. Here." He shows me a holographic picture of the man. "Get it done and I can guarantee your ticket off here."

I don't trust the Rat but what choice do I have?

Cooped up on long flights people don't always get along, especially those on Corporate dime. Most don't have the luxury of doing anything about it. It fascinates me just how much time, energy and money is spent on just making other people play nice.

I make my way to the barracks and thankfully the walls of the buildings along the way have been scoured clean of Holoads so nothing pops up to attract attention. I have had my fill of them for one day.

I keep my head down so I don't catch anybody's eye. It's common for people to come and go around the base so it doesn't have any checkpoints. Everyone on this rock is here for largely the same reasons and those who aren't everyone knows about soon enough. Corporate HQ never spends more money than is absolutely necessary, so I have no problem simply walking in.

The barracks are Corporation Standard. The Chief of Security's room is at the end of the corridor. I knock on the door and I yell that I have an urgent message from the docks but no one answers. I try a couple more times but there is no response.

I quickly look around before I pull out a universal lock decoder. It'll work on a standard issue door like this, the firmware is most likely seriously out of date so it should present no problem. The thing whirrs and I have it unlocked in less than a second.

Inside the place is a wreck. There are signs of a struggle, stuff is scattered all over the place. A bottle of something lies on the floor broken and, next to it there is a body, also broken and still. That Rat! He set me up. That mother f...

I can already hear voices coming down the corridor so my guess is the door was monitored. Some sort of trip-lock switch.

I have no time to come up with a better plan. I lock the door behind me and attach the decoder to the lock its settings turned to 'scramble'. It should buy me some time before they decide to break the door down. I quickly look around. The Chief's pass is on the floor, lying under his body. It should give me access to the cargo hold at the very least but I still have to make it out of here alive.

I open the cabin window, activate the powergrip on my boots and step out. I will have to climb all the way down to the next level.

The unmistakable noise of an oxy-torch being lit on the other side lets me know that I'd better not waste any more time.

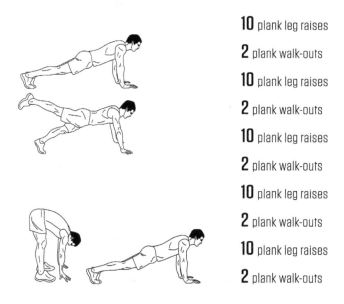

10 plank leg raises

2 plank walk-outs

10 plank leg raises

2 plank walk-outs

10 plank leg raises

2 plank walk-outs

10 plank leg raises

2 plank walk-outs

10 plank leg raises

2 plank walk-outs

It's not my lucky day.

The oxy-torch they used must have been industrial grade because I am only halfway down as a couple of heads pop up at the top. They spot me immediately and the bastards open fire.

In the rain, shooting downwards is not the easiest thing to do. Still, with my luck, right now I can take no chances.

I now have to climb and avoid the oncoming blasts.

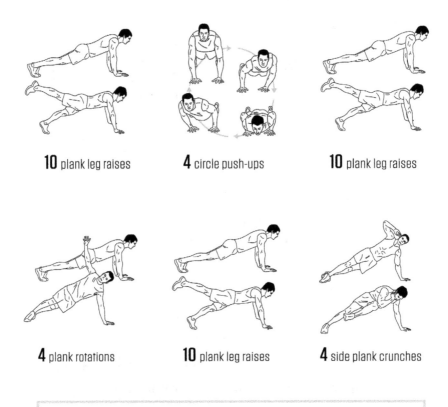

10 plank leg raises   **4** circle push-ups   **10** plank leg raises

4 plank rotations   **10** plank leg raises   **4** side plank crunches

catch your breath, rest up to 2 minutes, and repeat the circuit
7 times in total

I am lucky there is no one waiting for me on the ground. If "lucky" applies to this situation at all.

I jump down -

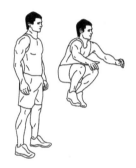

one jump knee tuck

and sprint for the docks.

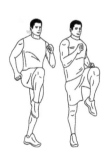

100 high knees

When I get there the Rat is nowhere to be seen. Which is probably a good thing since I really don't have time to deal with him and when I do it won't be pleasant. I can hear the engines beginning to fire up.

I use the Security Chief's pass I took from the room to get into the cargo hold and lock the door behind me. Moments later I hear the final seal being activated on the door. Talking about cutting it close!

It's a standard safety protocol: the doors will now be sealed until we get to the Hub. And after that, none of this will matter. I throw my stuff down and slide down against the door. Finally, I can rest. It's been a long night and I can't believe it's finally over. In seconds, I fall asleep.

Chapter 3

I wake up to the sound of gunfire and people screaming.
My brain is fuzzy from sleep but I have been here before. I
know the signs and noises and sounds and their meaning.
My brain filters out the dream from the reality. I realize with
clarity that the ship is under attack. My heart rate speeds
up, I take deep breaths. Not a dream. The ship really is
under attack and just like that I am completely awake and
functioning. Under attack. Great!

It's not uncommon for cargo ships to be attacked by pirates
in open space but it's usually the independent traders that
find themselves boarded and looted. It almost never happens
with corporate shipments and when it does, it's the pirates
that pay for their exercise of poor judgement - when they
are hunted down afterwards, caught and publicly executed

by being made to take a spacewalk without a suit. You don't screw with corporate stuff, everyone knows that. And if you do, you'd better make sure there is no trace left afterwards for anyone to find otherwise your goose is cooked.

Which means that whatever is happening on the ship - it's really bad news. It's only a matter of time until whoever is rampaging out there makes their way to where all the good stuff is: the cargo hold. I am guessing they are busy taking out the security staff right about now...

I guessed correctly. Someone stops right outside the door minutes later. I can hear muffled voices, someone giving orders and something being attached to the door on the other side... a precision explosive. I duck for cover behind one of the crates and after a dull thump the door falls off its hinges. All one hundred tons of it.

Five heavily armed men in high tech black uniforms step in guns at the ready all holding battle-ready formation. The leader gives the signal to spread out.

I can make out RIM Corp insignia on their armor and I dry swallow.

Regulators. RIM Corp are highly trained operatives with the latest nano-tech gear and by the looks of it they have just taken over the ship. Judging by the screams whatever they are doing here does not allow for leaving any witnesses behind.

Regardless, RIM Corp and I have a bad track record of getting along. I'd better figure something out before they find me.

My infrared blocker is always on, a precaution I've learned the hard way, so they can't pick me up on their scanners. As far as they can see on their screens the cargo hold has no warm bodies. I may not get an opportunity like this again to take out the whole group.

I move from crate to crate and keep low so I can isolate my targets and take them out one by one.

complete in any order, up to 2 minutes rest in between

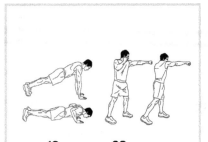

10 push-ups + **30** punches
repeat the combo 5 times in total
catch your breath in between if necessary

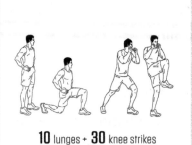

10 lunges + **30** knee strikes
repeat the combo 5 times in total
catch your breath in between if necessary

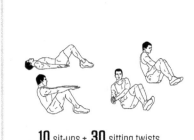

10 sit-ups + **30** sitting twists
repeat the combo 5 times in total
catch your breath in between if necessary

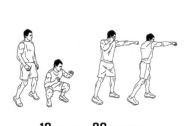

10 squats + **30** punches
repeat the combo 5 times in total
catch your breath in between if necessary

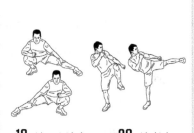

10 side-to-side lunges + **30** side kicks
repeat the combo 5 times in total
catch your breath in between if necessary

You don't get to be who I am without picking up a few handy interpersonal skills along the way. It's clean, bloodless work and within a few minutes I find myself lowering the last one, gently to the floor.

With him out of the way the imminent threat of being discovered is past. But I can't stay here, it's no longer safe. It'll be better if I make my way to the control deck and check for survivors. And I need to be ready in case there are more of them out there. And if Regulators are involved, this is not the end of it. I wonder what I got myself into exactly. This is supposed to be a routine flight, it's why I chose it as my ticket off GT-701.

What did I miss?

Chapter 4

My eyes are busy surveying the scene, taking in the damage, deciding the metadata to show me what happened here. It looks like the crew put up one hell of a fight but they never stood a chance against Regulators.

There is never a lot of security on corporate cargo ships and even then it's just a required check box. Something someone has to fill in. They never see any real action. So I was surprised there were trained men on board at all, anyone even capable of responding to gunfire.

I see several bodies on my way to the control deck. All of them precision kills but with some hesitation judging by the body positioning. It doesn't look like anyone from the crew survived. It is a massacre.

The deck itself has taken some damage from the attack too. I can smell something burning and there are sparks pouring from several blast holes all over. Preserving ship's function was not on the list of the Regulators' priorities it seems which makes this not just a planned attack but a planned attack that's designed to leave no evidence behind.

Regulators are corporate muscle. Highly trained, highly motivated, highly effective. I got lucky in the Hold because they were not expecting anyone. Taking on Regulators however is the easiest way to erase your existence.

I am working and I am thinking. Regulators attacking this ship makes no sense at all. This is Corporate property. They own it. Attacking it is not about gaining access to its cargo, at least not in the conventional sense. Something is going on here which I don't understand and now it really bugs me.

Things you fail to understand create blindspots. Blindspots get you killed. There's an elemental brutality in the simplicity of that equation that I admire as much as I detest. This is, maybe, not quite the future our ancestors had hoped for. Then again who can say with any degree of certainty and reading any kind of History of the origin planet leaves one feeling that maybe things are not quite so bad. It's one reason I don't read Histories. They make me feel jaded and that's an occupational hazard for me.

I shake my head to clear my thoughts and go straight to the control panel and check the system out for damage. I don't know what I am hoping for. Luck maybe? But luck is not on my side. It's really bad, the navigation system is down. I crack open the shielding and sure enough, some of the wiring is done for. I can probably salvage the parts if I look around but looking around is going to take time and maybe time is not what I have on my side.

I download the ship's schematics from the deck and bring it up in the hand-held projector on my wrist. There are several places I can try and see if I get lucky with what I need.

I check Medical first. It's called a Medical Bay but on a ship like this it is subject to the same pressure of not occupying payable space as everything else. So it is basically a closet with a few supplies but it's worth a shot. The door is blocked from the inside but I can probably get in through the vents. I check the schematics again to confirm. There is indeed access through one of the service vents so crawling through the vents it is then.

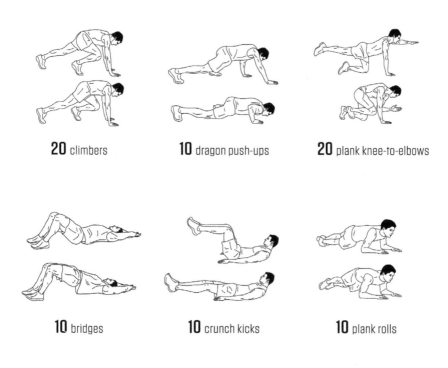

20 climbers   **10** dragon push-ups   **20** plank knee-to-elbows

10 bridges   **10** crunch kicks   **10** plank rolls

catch your breath, rest up to 2 minutes, and repeat the circuit
7 times in total

I jump down and look through the supplies. There is nothing I can use in here, unfortunately. This ship's Medical is more paired down than usual. I unblock the door from the debris that had been preventing it from opening and I walk out.

Some cargo ships have smaller emergency control panels in the Captain cabins for remote operations. This ship doesn't seem to be nearly advanced enough but I still need to make sure. As I walk in, I realize the gravity in this room is out of whack. It seems to fluctuate from spot to spot making searching the room a bit of a challenge as half of it floats up in the air. I'll have to move around the furniture using my grip-boost boots and even push some of it out of the way.

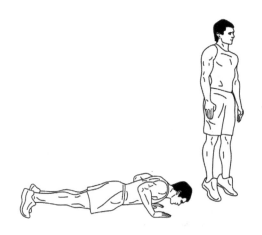

10 burpees

catch your breath

10 burpees

catch your breath

10 burpees

catch your breath

10 burpees

catch your breath

10 burpees

My gambit pays off! Maybe my luck isn't quite as bad as I think it is after all. I find what I want floating in the middle of the cabin. After some effort and a little gyrating in zero G, I grab the planshet from the air and take my bounty back to the control deck.

After a little work the system is back up and running. Now, let's see...

"Computer, what's our current location?"

"Solar Luna-5" - a pleasant female voice responds.

"Resume course."

"Resuming course to Andromeda 6."

"Hmm, no, that can't be right. Computer, set course to Hub-1."

"Changing course to Hub-1."

As the system confirms the new course, I hear a voice behind me shout: "No!"

I am not alone.

Chapter 5

"We must continue on this course!"

A small white haired girl continues to scream at me. Her hair is ash-blonde to the point of appearing grey. I don't think she is older than twelve, if I was to guess. And she is probably still in shock surviving all of this. She must have walked past dead bodies and burnt out bulkheads to get to here.

"I need to go to Andromeda 6! Please!"

"Look, kid, whoever you are, I don't care where you want to go but this ship is going to Hub-1."

"My name is Ellie, not kid. And you are…"

I am guessing she just now realized I wasn't a crew member. She must have been watching me for a while to determine that I am not a Regulator but not long enough to see I am not part of this ship's staff either. I smirk.

She backs towards the wall. I can tell she is not armed and she doesn't move like someone used to combat. I quickly assess she is no immediate threat to me.
"Don't worry, I am not with the other guys as you can see. I am the off-manifest guest."

"Oh."

She seems to relax a little bit but is still staying on the other side of the room, as far away from me as she get. It's probably smart, too, since I haven't decided what to do with her yet. If I was one of the Regulators she would be a pile of red dust right now. Then again… that would simplify things.

I decide to clarify things for the both of us: "Alright, listen. We are going to Hub-1 and you can hitchhike anywhere you want from there. You mind your own business and I'll mind my own. We will not have a problem."

I can tell this is not what she wants to hear but I am not giving her much of a choice. She swallows hard and then slowly nods. It's good enough for me.

"Splendid," she mumbles, but I ignore that. I have no time for playing games or building any kind of relationship beyond the strictly functional required by the moment.
I turn around to face the control panel and start a diagnostic sequence. It'll take some time, these things are complex. I glance back to make sure the girl is still there... A-a-and she's gone.

Dammit, I didn't even hear her move! She is going to be a problem after all. Swearing silently to myself for my stupidity I dash after her.

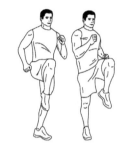

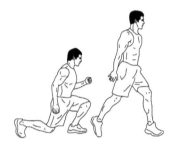

20 high knees

2 jumping lunges

20 high knees

2 jumping lunges

20 high knees

2 jumping lunges

20 high knees

2 jumping lunges

20 high knees

2 jumping lunges

catch your breath, rest up to 2 minutes, and repeat the circuit
7 times in total

Chapter 6

The problem with cargo ships is that they're functional.
There are corridors and tunnels and entrance ways. Service
tubes and access hatches and control panel points. Because
the cargo hold is their reason for being everything revolves
around the cargo hold and everything is done to maximize
its space and minimize everything else, no matter how vital it
might be.

Corporate shareholder mentality at its best.

This creates a maze of corridors to anyone not familiar with a cargo ship's layout. And because no cargo ship is the same the maze of passages and corridors is always unique which is a clever way of saying you can get lost up there if you're not careful. Or you could lose someone.

I tell myself I am, right now, in the latter group. Great!

Did she turn this way?... Damn, the kid is fast.

I take a wild guess and choose the passage most likely to appeal to a scared young girl. It's one that leads to the cargo hold, though, to be fair - from a certain point of view all corridors and passages on a cargo ship lead to the cargo hold. It's just ahead and there is no other way out.

I speed up to get there faster. I get to the door and every sense I have makes me freeze.

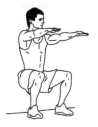

60 Seconds wall sit

I can hear voices. Distant. Metallic. Comms tones. Possibly military judging by the clipped sentences.

"Package acquired. Over."

"Roger that. We have your coordinates locked. We'll pick you up shortly, hold tight."

There are two of them. Both Regulators, both heavily armed and looking alert. One of them is handling something. I see a little body lying on the floor nearby. The girl's arms and legs are secured with electro-bonds so she must still be alive.

I guess she ran in there to hide from me and that's when they grabbed her.

"How are we doing with the explosives?"

"This stuff is delicate. I'll need some time."

"Well, hurry then, the extraction team are on their way." Explosives? Great! They are going to blow up the ship and me along with it. I have to do something and fast before their friends arrive. I don't have time to think of something more strategic so I will have to take them both head on.

When the element of surprise is on your side you have a decided advantage. Trained or not the Regulators didn't think anyone else was alive on the ship besides them and the girl they'd captured. It was a mistake that would cost them, as it turned out.

I picked the moment when they were both absorbed with their equipment and its writing and came out of my hiding.

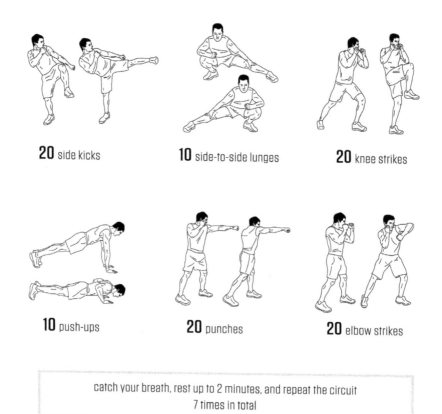

20 side kicks   **10** side-to-side lunges   **20** knee strikes

10 push-ups   **20** punches   **20** elbow strikes

catch your breath, rest up to 2 minutes, and repeat the circuit
7 times in total

Now, for the other problem...

Chapter 7

I brought the girl, I think she said Ellie was her name, back to the control room. I decided to keep the electro-bonds The Regulators put on her until I am sure she won't run again. She's regained consciousness a while back as I was carrying her, but she's pretending she hasn't. She is not as stupid as she looks but then neither am I.

I am the first to break the silence: "I know you are awake. If I wanted to hurt you I would have done that already. At this moment, I am no danger to you. Nod if you understand." She opens her eyes, looks straight at me and nods.

"So now that we have that established we have a problem. Two, in fact, and one of them is more pressing than the other. The guys who were after you, well, bad news - there are more of them coming. They seem to want you alive. It's a wild guess but judging by all the explosive they were setting up, I don't think they are planning on leaving any evidence behind. And yet, this is not the worst news." I pause to let my words sink in, then continue: "See this bar here, flashing red?"

She nods again.

"These are our oxygen reserves. When these guys took over the ship they must have damaged the generators. It wouldn't be so bad but it looks like we also have a leak. The levels wouldn't be dropping this fast otherwise. We are running out of air and fast. By my estimation we have maybe an hour, an hour and a half left at best. I could just throw you into the airlock and buy myself more time... Don't get me wrong, you seem like a nice kid and all but I don't owe you anything. That said, I don't know how much time I need and if it'll be enough so I am being honest here. My proposition is simple: I work alone and maybe I make it or we work together and we both make it. I'll need more than a nod this time."

"You are not a very nice person." She says.

"I am the nicest one around. Do you want to live or not?"

"I do. What do you need me to do?"

"I can seal the leak to buy us more time but I would have to do it from the outside. This is a type-C cargo ship, the only way in is if someone lets you in. I will make sure we don't die from suffocation, or at least raise our chances so we don't die from suffocation in the next hour, and you make sure I can get back inside."

"What stops me from just leaving you out there after you fix the leak?"

"The same thing that stops me from making a new hole in this ship: self-preservation. We will have to work together for the time being so both of us can survive."

"Alright then. You can take these off now." She nods to her electro-bonds.

I free the girl and we go over the plan one more time. Her part is relatively easy, she just has to let me back in once I am done, but it's going to be tricky for me on the outside. All cargo ships have emergency gear for space walks but it's usually badly maintained - if at all. I'll be lucky if my suit holds. What's the alternative, though? Sure suffocation in here or a likely suffocation out there. Who said the universe was not a big gamble? They were lying and probably knew nothing of Heisenberg for whom the entire cosmos was a matter of degrees of uncertainty calculated within certain relational values to each other.

"Hold on to this for me."

I give her one of the comms I took from the Regulators. I then put on a suit, take a really deep breath to acclimate my lungs to the pressure and step into the airlock.

Decompression... My suit suddenly becomes my lifeboat. Air and pressure leach away fast: 98%... 99%... 100%... here we go. One foot in front of the other.

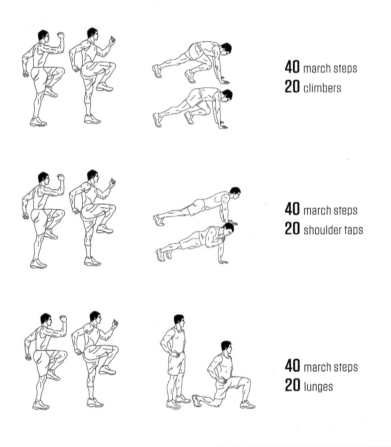

40 march steps
20 climbers

40 march steps
20 shoulder taps

40 march steps
20 lunges

catch your breath, rest up to 2 minutes, and repeat the circuit
7 times in total

I get to the damaged side of the ship and start working on the crack I see there. At least from the outside things are easier to spot. It doesn't take me long to fix it – the Lords of Mirth are looking out for us. If the crack was any bigger we would have already been dead. There, done. I have to make it all the way back now and hope that the kid holds up her end of the deal.

She should ... but...

I make it back and I am beginning to feel light-headed as the last reserves of oxygen in the suit are beginning to run out... The airlock is just ahead of me however, one more step... I get there, and the door is still locked. I begin to feel the tight pain as my chest constricts, diaphragm gasping for breath. I try to regulate my heartbeat, control the rising sense of dread and panic. My brain feels sluggish and there are dark spots dancing in front of my eyes and then the closing down of the world; as tunnel vision shuts down my sight into a single bright, circular spot of very bright white light.

Damn.

Chapter 8

GASP! I am gulping for air as someone takes my helmet off. My vision is still blurry from the pressure and my chest kinda aches but I am beginning to see clearer now and there is no sharp pain in my lungs to deal with so I agues I am not dying. At least not just yet. Ellie is kneeling in front of me, her eyes are wide. I struggle to orient myself.

"I am so sorry! I panicked! You suddenly stopped moving and I didn't know what to do. You were close enough for me to reach but I wasn't suited up. It took time for me to put one on and drag you back in."

I frown.

"It was incredibly stupid."

And brave though I do not tell her that. Overall, though, really stupid. She could have just left me there to die. Once the oxygen ran out I would have been as helpless as a kitten out there. She looks terrified. Does she think I am going to hurt her now? No, not me.

"They're coming. The comms started transmitting when you were out. They will be here any minute."

"We should hurry then."

I nod towards the cargo hold.

"We can use the uniforms from those two and wait for the arrival. This ship is not going to last much longer so we need to ditch it. And whoever is after you is about to give us a way out."

We both hurry to the cargo hold and find the uniforms of the dead Regulators. It's nanotech so it adjusts to the size of the body. Once we are geared up no one will see our faces. We should be able to blend in. We might just pull it off.

We don't need to wait long. The comms start transmitting again.

"Zeta Team, come in. This is Destroyer-1. Where are you guys? Over."

"Yes, Destroyer-1. Ready for pick up. Over."

"Roger that. ETA 45 minutes. End of transmission."
I turn to Ellie.

"We can't have them question us so we need a diversion. I am going to use their own explosives and set several charges around the place. Once they open the doors a few small detonations should distract them enough for us to make our way in. I'll get on it now."

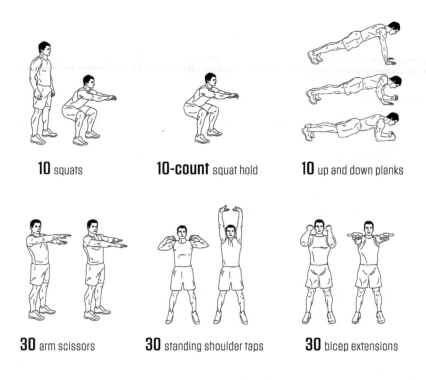

10 squats   10-count squat hold   10 up and down planks

30 arm scissors   30 standing shoulder taps   30 bicep extensions

catch your breath, rest up to 2 minutes, and repeat the circuit
7 times in total

That's it, that's the last one. And just in time, too, they are
here. I wave to Ellie to open the shaft for the ship to fly in. A
black Destroyer makes its way inside the ship's landing dock.
It engages the booster rockets cushioning its landing, aligns
itself with the guide lights in the landing bay and lands.
The doors open and we see several men in black uniforms
running towards us.

It's all a matter of timing.

"NOW!"

I yell and I detonate the explosives. There is the dull thud of explosive compounds consuming oxygen and expanding rapidly in a pressurized environment and then the deck underfoot trembles in a way that indicates that something is very wrong with the ship. It's time to run.

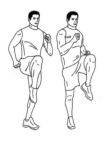

100 high knees

In the confusion the men freeze on the spot for a second or two. No one shoots. They wait for us to get closer and then close in behind us. We all run inside locking the doors.

"It's all going to blow! Go, go, go! Take off, NOW!"

The pilot doesn't waste time and takes off as the cargo ship starts exploding right underneath us. We just make it out as the whole place goes up in flames. This stuff was a lot, a LOT more potent than I thought. It must be a new compound if it can vaporize an entire cargo ship with no trace left with just a few charges. I dry swallow at the prospect of turning into dust along with it.

I turn to the Regulators now surrounding us both thinking that in running the scenario in my head I had miscalculated a few variables.

"So, it's a funny story." I begin and someone strikes me from behind with something hard, on the back of the head.

Chapter 9

We were restrained within seconds. I was unconscious. They collared us regardless and threw us both into a holding cell. I was kicked a few times for good measure, too. One of the men pulled out a bio scanner and scanned our implants.

"Yep, identity confirmed. That's Eleonora Ri. And this one here is a nobody as far as I can tell. I recommend a quick execution to be prudent."

"Captain Jackal wanted to deal with this personally. Our first priority right now is to make sure the ship hasn't been damaged with all of the fireworks and once I have men to spare I want these two watched until we get back to base."

They left us alone.

I try my collar and get a jolt of pain. Advanced tech that
reads mental waves like a mini, portable fMRI. You even
think of escaping you get an electric shock to set you straight.
I look around the hold and check it for weaknesses. There
are none that I can see. I need to think so I drop down on the
floor.

"What the hell are you doing?"

"Push-Ups. It helps me think."

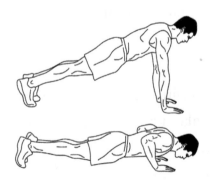

10 push-ups

catch your breath

10 push-ups

catch your breath

10 push-ups

catch your breath

10 push-ups

catch your breath

10 push-ups

I work up a good sweat, sit down in the corner opposite Ellie and turn to face her.

"So, what do they want with you anyway? Just so I know what I am dealing with here. At least they want you alive but I am on borrowed time here."

She sighed.

"How much do you know about Xelium mining?"
"As much as anyone else. It's incredibly potent fuel and it's fairly easy to mine. Most of the GT planets have it. It's a simple extraction process provided you have the Corp money behind you for the equipment. The Corporations have a stranglehold on this, maintaining a monopoly that keeps prices artificially stable and fuel available everywhere planets play nice. Have I missed out anything?"

"Not bad. Well, there's a little more to it. It's in growing demand whereas GT planets are getting further and further away. The more you mine, the more you need. The further the planet, the lesser the profit. Transports already take longer and longer so the Corporations are beginning to hike up the price.

Something that was as common as dirt yesterday is going to get as precious as gold tomorrow. My father explained it all to me."

I think for a minute. Xelium indeed used to be as common as dirt - everyone could get hold of it. Without specialized equipment large-scale production was impossible, but it could be mined even in backwater planets using 20th Century tech. Within a hundred years there has never been a shortage or any trouble of getting a fairly reasonable supply that would last you long enough to cross the Galaxy and you'll still have enough left for a return journey. It's what made space exploration possible - and accessible to all. With time Xelium started getting more and more expensive and these days solo transports no longer exist. It's too expensive, you need to have the backing of someone, or even better, you need to be sponsored directly by a Corp, to cover any significant distances. Indeed, come to think of it even GT-701 did not produce nearly enough to justify it having a colony.

"OK, but what does it have to do with you?"

"My father was working for the RIM Corp, he was looking into ways of improving Xelium extraction. You know, squeeze more out of the deposits and such? Then something changed. He became secretive at first and then he grew more and more paranoid... Eventually, one day he just sent me away saying it was no longer safe for me to remain with him. He told me it broke his heart but he would never forgive himself if something was to happen to me. He arranged a transport for me with a one-way ticket to GT-701. He promised he'll get me the moment he could. And then two weeks ago I got a message from my uncle that it was no longer safe for me and that he'd arranged a transport for me to come to Andromeda 6."

Her eyes start watering.

"He said he thought my father was dead and he told me to trust no one and stay hidden".

She wiped tears off her cheeks with her sleeves.

"That's solid advice right there."

Suddenly said someone from the other side of the room. The empty other side of the room.

Chapter 10

The man the voice belonged to, introduced himself as Reed, the infamous Grand Hacker. I'd never heard of him.

"As I was saying, I was minding my own business here when the two of you joined me. It was incredibly inconvenient, you know. Even more so when these guys took off without any warning. I figured this will be the perfect place to hide."

"How come we didn't see you before?"

"Oh that, I have a personal cloaking field. It's something I designed for an emergency like this actually. I have to stand very still for it to work, though, and it takes a while to kick in and blend with the surroundings but otherwise, a brilliant tool. I was listening to you two and you seemed like an alright pair. I figured it was safe to come out. Plus, if they are going to bring more people in here it'll get super crowded. I did the math and well, hello."

"If you don't mind me asking, ahem, what were you doing here to begin with. You don't look like a Regulator, which is no criticism, you understand."

"I was trying to steal the ship, naturally. You know how much someone will pay for a Destroyer on the black market?" - he whistles to himself.

I glance at Ellie and even she looks terrified.

"Sure, messing with the Corp property is going to be incredibly rewarding."

Reed doesn't seem phased in the least. He just brushes it off.

"That's what makes it so valuable, there aren't any for sale. The reward justifies the risk. Just like talking to you guys, in my opinion, it justifies the risk of you turning me in right now. You won't do that, though, right?"

"You said you were a hacker. Can you deal with these?"

I point at our cell and the collars.

"Yes and no. I can disable the safeguards so you could take the collars off but the cell functions run at a frequency that'll instantly sent out an alert if tampered with. The same with the collars. The moment you take them off, boom - all seven, I counted seven, Regulators rush in here guns blazing. No-no-no, I don't do guns and dying. A firm no to dying."

"Fair enough. No to dying. Rendering the safeguards useless is already something. I can work with that."

I explain my plan to Reed and Ellie and we agree to work together. It takes a few minutes for Reed to deactivate the safeguards. Watching him work I couldn't help but be impressed. The man himself has clearly been heavily modified with most of his tech being directly implanted into his nervous system. I've heard of extreme modifications like that but I've never met a hypermod in person before. You don't usually meet them in the street to be fair - they are notorious hermits as they don't trust anyone or anything but tech. Reed is indeed something.

After the job was done, Reed hid just like he did before so it was just me and Ellie in the cell as far as anyone could see. About an hour later two Regulators come down to the cells, they both have their visors down but otherwise they have their full gear on. A man and a woman.

The woman goes to sit by the door, clearly preoccupied with something else on her screen. And the man comes closer to the holding cell to take a better look at us. They're busy talking to each other.

"Ridiculous assignment, we are the best of the best and here we are fetching and watching. It's beneath us."

"Just chill out, it's not so bad."

"You are just happy you can stare at your comics all day."

"Graphic Novels. And yeah, I don't mind that. I get to catch up on the latest issue of the Red Reaper. Man, they don't make them like that anymore."

"It's trash. Honestly, for a professional operative you really do like these fairy tales."

"They are not fairy tales, the Red Reaper is a legend. Do you know the killcount? No one does. Some say it might be tens of thousands. Just the Orion massacre comes to a total of 5,000. They say they had to shovel through red dust just to get to the base there was just nothing left. And that was all just one man."

"Yeah, right. I bet if I met him he would piss his pants."

"Why do you think the Reaper is a man? Could have been a woman, too, no one can say for sure."

"Regardless, it's all a pile of crap anyway. Look at these two in here, - he pointed at me and Ellie, - a waste of space and our time, too. We lost two teams down there and these two make it? I want to know how."

I perk up at the opportunity. Curiosity isn't a sin but it really should be. I've seen entire squads decimated in action because a member couldn't resist their curiosity and did something they shouldn't. Cats, folklore tells us, know this well. But they still can't resist poking their noses where they're likely to use up some of their nine lives. People, really, don't stand a chance. Far fewer than nine lives, you see.

"You can come in here and ask me." I say.

"Now, why would I do that?" says the man.

He presses something on his wrist and I get a powerful jolt of pain spreading from the collar through my entire body. The pain is excruciating, I drop down on the floor, convulsing. Part of me sees in my mind what I must look like and it ain't a pretty picture. I hate him already but I control it. The part of my brain where all the secret bad things hide in is seething with anger and a clear voice whispers in its darkness: here kitty, kitty, kitty.

"That all you got?" I gasp through gritted teeth.

I get another jolt. And I can see from the corner of my eye panic spreading through Ellie's face.

"Now," - I spit out blood, - "It's not as satisfying, is it? Pushing buttons is hardly manly. You were boasting about taking on the Reaper just moments ago and you are afraid to get your hands dirty."

He takes the bait. The force field around us vanishes as he disables it through the remote on his wrist.

Then, he goes for me. Kitty. Kitty. Kitty.

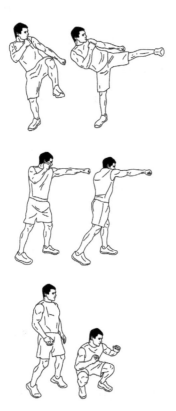

20 side kicks

20 punches

one squat

20 side kicks

20 punches

one squat

20 side kicks

20 punches

one squat

20 side kicks

20 punches

one squat

His friend in the corner, engrossed with her Graphic Novel, was not paying attention to our fight until it was too late. She clearly relied on the safety of the collars to get me back into line at any point and was just letting her partner release some steam.

Fortunately for me and unfortunately for her what happened next was too fast for her to even reach for her remote.

It's easy to hold back when it's just practice, when it's a show. When it's life and death something very primal kicks in. Something raw and powerful rises up to the surface. All this time I was trying to get him to position just right, in a very specific spot...

With a quick upward elbow strike I knock out the guy's teeth and duck. Simultaneously, Reed unclips my collar and clips it to the Regulator's neck. It was the signal to Ellie, who I knew only too well was a mistake to misjudge and who was lightning fast. She does the same with the neck of the female Regulator - minus knocking out her teeth.

In moments, both Regulators are in our places, disabled and collared. And we are free to do what we have to do.

Chapter 11

Reed had no problem unlocking the Regulators' weapons for me but he refused to handle any himself. I even got one of their handy wrist controls. I check the gun and instantly feel sick. It's a pulverizer. I've heard that they became more popular amongst corporate goons but I hoped it was just rumors. They were outlawed under the penalty of death across the Galaxy... I sigh.

Those who control the law are the law. And often it does not apply to them. My hand with a gun in it shook a little at the thought of the damage this thing could do. Memories ... I remember ...

"Are you alright?" - asked Ellie noticing my hesitation.

"Yeah, it's ok. Bad memories, that is all. So, I think we are all agreed, we need to return the favor and take over the ship. We can't let them take us to their Command base. No way we are getting out of the HQ alive. Which brings us to the present problem - the five more Regulators onboard. We are lucky this is a small ship with a minimal crew so the three of us...," - I look at the kid and the geek. "So I can probably handle the rest of them. We will need to lure them in, though, unlike with the cargo ship where they didn't care whether it stays intact we actually care about preserving this transport. I can't use the guns in the control deck, the chances of damaging the controls are too high. We need to lure them, preferably one at a time. Which is where you two come in."

I come up with a plan where Reed and Ellie will cause distractions around the ship to separate the Regulators and eventually make them come down here. Ellie will use her weasel-like speed and lure one of them first. She has an advantage - they want her unharmed so she is pretty safe.

And Reed will mess with their comms to make them think there is a problem down here.

To give me an advantage I decide to move a few things around to create cover. It's been a long time since I held a gun and I couldn't tell for sure if I would be able to use it. I didn't share those fears with the other two. What they need right now is someone in control or we will all fall apart.

There is no time for doubts. I begin to move the furniture and pile things up.

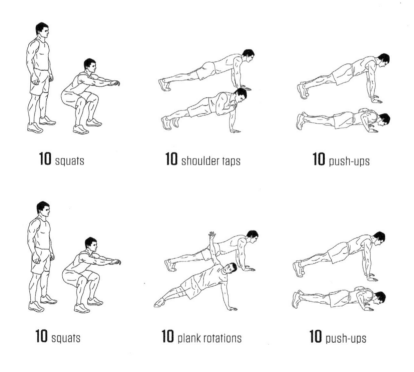

10 squats   10 shoulder taps   10 push-ups

10 squats   10 plank rotations   10 push-ups

catch your breath, rest up to 2 minutes, and repeat the circuit
7 times in total

We agree on the ETA and I only have a few minutes left by the time I finish. I brace myself and take the position. It's not long before the first Regulator comes in through the door.

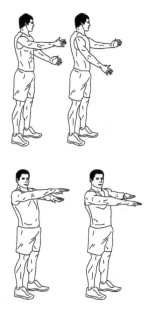

keep arms up throughout

20 scissor chops

10 arm scissors

20 scissor chops

10 arm scissors

20 scissor chops

10 arm scissors

20 scissor chops

10 arm scissors

20 scissor chops

10 arm scissors

By the time I've dealt with the last of them, both my hands were beginning to shake and I had to pull myself together for my new crew's sake.

Killing has never been a problem for me but killing with vaporizers... It is a whole different story. Erasing people into dust, the ease and speed with which it happens, that's what bothers me. Taking a life should not be so easy, so final, so... soulless. Erasing someone from existence and leaving but an empty heap of grain behind. It's something I hoped I could never see again much less do myself.

All that is left from the five Regulators, except the two in the holding cell, are five piles of red dust and their gear. Vaporizers target carbon-based bodies only, leaving everything else intact. It disintegrates a person, everything they were and may have been. Poof, and you are gone like you've never existed before.

Still, it is not the time nor the place to have these thoughts. I take a deep breath and turn to Reed and Ellie, both of whom have now come down to the Holding cell and are standing next to me looking relieved we are no longer in immediate danger. Am I the only one concerned with so much death?

Why does it follow me everywhere I go? Will it ever stop?
"Reed, I assume you can fly this thing. Take us somewhere
safe." I say and my voice is unusually tight, even for me.

Chapter 12

"So," Reed continues, "it'll take some time to change our engine signature. In the meantime we will hide in the asteroid noise. They won't be able to pick our signal out as long as we stay amongst the rocks. They provide excellent interference!"

We got lucky to come across this debris. This must have been a star at one point or another and now it's just rocks, a lot of them. Broken and scattered they still stayed somewhat together creating the perfect curtain for us to hide behind. We went in as far as we could and "parked" the Destroyer on the largest rock we could find.

I notice Ellie looking out in fascination.

"Pretty, isn't it?"

"Yeah, - she responds without taking her eyes off the view, - I've never seen a formation like that before."

"I lived near a very similar one as a kid. - I say. - It was my very own playground. As a matter of fact... Hey, Reed, how long did you say you'll need to change the signature?"

"Mmmm, about an hour. There is a lot of manual work involved since I can't connect to the network. The block works both ways, you see"

"Yeah-yeah, alright. I don't need to know the details. You don't need us here to do any of this, though, right?"

"No-o-ope."

"Perfect. Ellie?"

I throw a nano-tech suit her way.

"Suit up. We are going for a walk."

Her face lights up for the first time since we met.

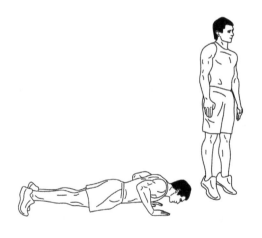

10 burpees

catch your breath

10 burpees

catch your breath

10 burpees

catch your breath

10 burpees

catch your breath

10 burpees

I can hear her laugh through the comms as we leap from rock to rock like a couple of frogs. For a second there even I forget all my worries. I've been so focused on survival, for such a long time now that I never had a spare moment to think about anything else. And here, in the endless space in the middle of nowhere I just suddenly feel at peace. I feel that perhaps I could just stay here forever, no longer be the hunter or the hunted...

"You know, I never even asked your name." - I hear Ellie say through the comms."

"It's Sef. You can call me Sef."

"Nice to meet you, Sef."

"Em? I hate to be a party-pooper but you'd better come back inside." - We hear Reed say through the comms. - "We've got company."

Chapter 13

We rush back in just as Reed fires up the engines of the Destroyer.

"What's going on, Reed?"

"They must have figured out we would hide here. I didn't have enough time to finish the signature swap. Another thirty minutes or so, that's all I needed … but there is no point now. They can see us. There are two Destroyers hailing us right now. So, any ideas anyone?"

"Run." - I say, - "They want Ellie, but they will not think twice over killing you and me, Reed. We have to give running a shot. They won't fire at us just yet so we might just have a shot."

"Alright. Let's see how fast this baby can go. "

He sounded way more excited than he had any right to be, but I was beginning to get used to Reed's peculiar nature so I ignored it.

"I wrote the code for the signature change, it'll just need to finish rendering. If we manage to lose them in the open space they won't be able to find us so easily again. I did find a possible escape route we could take when scanning the area but it's... well, risky to say the least."

"What is it, just spit it out."

"There is a registered wormhole only ten minute from here. It's one of the unstable ones. There is no saying where we will pop out, if at all. Or if we are going to have all our limbs intact."

"Are you freaking kidding me..."

"By my calculations, we won't be able to outrun the Destroyers and there are two of them so... you do the math. We don't have sufficient firepower and I am not yet as familiar with the controls. This baby is advanced."

"Alright. Ellie, are you ok with this? We could hand you over before we take the leap if you think you have higher survival chances with the Regulators. After all, they do want you alive. I feel like at the very least I should ask."

"No. Even if they do now, they will torture and then most likely kill me anyway. Besides, you have better chances of making it to the wormhole with me onboard. They will have no problem shooting you down once they have me. We are in this together now."

"Reed?"

"I am onboard with not dying. Definitely dying and maybe dying, not so much. I'll take those odds. I am setting the course now but there is something else I need you to do."

"Ok, What is it?"

"Our chances are higher if we moved all the heavy stuff away from the control room. You know, just in case. Everything you can possibly rip away and get rid of and fast. We will not be in control while we are going through so anything can happen during that time."

"I am on it. Ellie, you sit tight."

I start moving everything away to the holding cell.

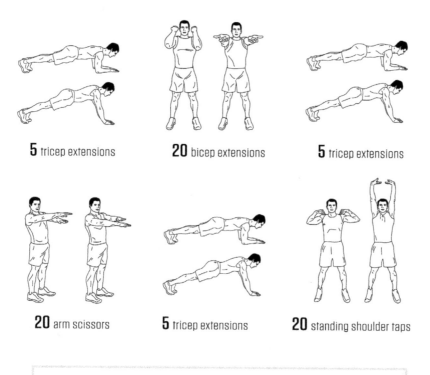

5 tricep extensions   **20** bicep extensions   **5** tricep extensions

20 arm scissors   **5** tricep extensions   **20** standing shoulder taps

catch your breath, rest up to 2 minutes, and repeat the circuit
7 times in total

"We are about to go in! The two destroyers are slowing down, I don't think they'll follow us! Brace your...."

Chapter 14

My lungs fill up with dust and I begin to cough. I am disoriented and my ears are ringing. I am on the ground and I can't see anything at all. It's all a blur. There are people. There are people running everywhere.

Another bomb goes off right next to me. It throws me back and here is that ringing again. I check for my blaster and it's not there. I start feeling the ground around me in hope it may have fallen somewhere nearby. A woman holding a child runs past and suddenly she gets hit in the back and disintegrates, crumbles into dust right in front of my eyes, the child rolls out of her arms as they crumble into red dust.

I see others, running and being shot.

I stay low. I can't get up, I won't get up. I begin to crawl as fast as I can.

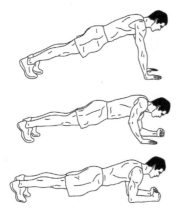

6 up and down planks

catch your breath

6 up and down planks

catch your breath

6 up and down planks

catch your breath

6 up and down planks

catch your breath

6 up and down planks

I see a chunk of metal, probably part of a ship, and I crawl to it for cover. I press my whole body against it and feel the cold and the burning. I can smell death, everywhere.

I see my gun, finally, there on the ground and I reach for it. I almost get it but someone steps on my hand, crushing it with a heavy boot.

"Stay down."

I look up and there is someone standing over me with a blaster pointed at my face.

"Any last words, you miserable piece of shit?"

I am tired. I am done. I am ready for this to be over. As I close my eyes, I brace myself and take what I imagine is my last breath when something light and fluffy begins to fall on my cheeks. What the... I open my eyes and I am covered in red dust. The man that stood over me is no more. I look past where he was standing and see the kid, the same kid the woman was carrying, with my blaster in his little hands, steaming.

The kid is in shock. Almost by instinct, I grab the blaster from his hands, pick up the kid and run.

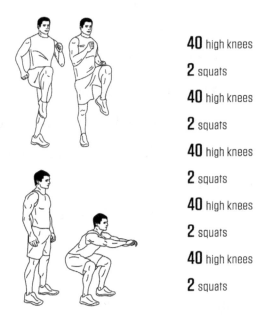

40 high knees

2 squats

40 high knees

2 squats

40 high knees

2 squats

40 high knees

2 squats

40 high knees

2 squats

Dust... red dust is everywhere. It covers everything as far as the eye can see. I can't make out anything at all. I just run. Any second now a blaster will go off somewhere and I will add to the endless sea of red...

"Sef! SEF!"

Someone is shaking me back into consciousness. The scene stretches out in front of me like an anomaly and then disintegrates and then there is Ellie standing over me. Her eyes are wide open. A worried Reed is right next to her with an expression of concern. Wormhole fever. I've heard of it. Well, now I have experienced it too. The brain cannot take the spacetime stretch without experiencing mini-psychotic episodes of its own. If you think that sounds bad, you're right.

I blink to clear my eyes. Try to sound nonchalant.

"I am ok."

I look around and I am still on board the Destroyer.

"Did we make it?"

"Yes."

I take a deep breath and fall back in my seat. I swear, I can still taste blood in my mouth.

Chapter 15

"It could have been worse."

"Worse? How?!"

"We could have landed in totally uncharted territory. This is at least known coordinates. Granted, it could have been better but, on the bright side, we are alive and we are not currently being pursued or fired upon."

"Yes, but we are literally in the middle of nowhere. How are we doing for fuel? It'll take us a substantial amount to get back to civilization."

"About that... We might be running low on Xelium."

I am beginning to get a headache. I put my fingers to my temples and attempt a massage. Just when I think the worst is over this stuff just keeps on happening. I find myself weirdly longing for an ad hologram to tell me again about Eden, the paradise. I shake it off by clamping down on my teeth. Bringing the sharp edges together. My tongue rubs against them and the sensation suddenly grounds me. Wormhole jumps are bad medicine. They can really mess with your head and mine has been messed with way more than average.

"Are there any occupied planets nearby? Outposts? Trading centers? Anything at all?"

Reed checks the charts and scratches the back of his head.

"There is a tribal planet a reasonable distance from here but there isn't much information on it. It's a GT-type planet so they should have Xelium. They may be willing to trade. Shall we go there? It's fully terraformed so we won't even need any extra gear."

"Do we have any other choice?" - I ask sarcastically.

Reed inputs the coordinates. He really is a man of no words, when interfacing with machines is an available option to him. I leave him to his task and go down to check on our Regulator prisoners.

To my annoyance, they are both alive and well and still restrained by the collars. They didn't try to escape as far as I can tell. I brought down a couple of bottles of water with me and pass them on to the woman.

"What is your name, Regulator?"

"Sam." - She replies after taking several gulps of water. Her partner refuses it. - "And his name is Raynar. Are you going to kill us? You must know Regulators don't negotiate for their own."

"I don't kill prisoners. Whoever they are. And I don't plan negotiating with your commanders either. Ideally I would like to drop you off somewhere convenient for me and inconvenient for you. As it happens, we might just be far enough from anywhere important so I will be able to do just that. Get ready, you are coming with me."

She seems to process it and nods to herself, seemingly relieved. Her partner just spits to the side. I don't care for his bravado. After all, it's the same man who had no problem beating me up when I was collared. I have no sympathy for him. I wait as they both get on their feet.

I return back to Reed and Ellie with the two Regulators trailing behind me. It looks like we have arrived at our destination and coming into range of the GT-type planet. Hopefully, we'll be able to trade with whomever inhabits it. The headache is still throbbing at the back of my head and I wonder whether hyperspace jumps do cumulative damage. There are rumors about that but no one has made enough jumps and been studied for data to exist on it and inanimate objects are no help here. I focus on the task at hand. Giving orders at least provides a distraction from the pain inside my head.

"We will drop off these two here. Reed, take us to the surface."

We make sure we land near a large habitat but not too close in case we freak out the natives. It unnerves me that we don't know much about this place. We have no idea what we are walking into.

Despite being a GT-type, it's a green planet. Why would someone terraform it this far away from literally anywhere? There is greenery everywhere; things buzzing in the air and crawling on the ground. There is blue sky and the sunlight is so bright, it really hurts my eyes.

Reed checks the holomap to see where the settlement is and points to the right. We'll have to cut through the vegetation. I make sure our prisoners go first so I can keep an eye on them.

We cut past the plants and trees and eventually come into the clearing. There are very basic huts all over it and people in patched up leather roaming about. It looks like a primitive village. I've heard about places like this, caught in a timewarp of their own cultural reticence. I had never seen one because … well, my travels in the past never took me near one. That's not quite where I had been needed. But now …

Reed did mention it was a tribal community, I just didn't realize it was this tribal. I look around in true fascination, all my senses suddenly alert.

It's not unusual for people to reject technology and form communities like this. After having seen first hand some of the worst excesses of the 'civilized' world a desire to escape from civilization is something I totally get. But there usually is still some civilization present. Some amenities that spell out progress. That is not what's going on here.

We are spotted by a bunch of kids and are instantly surrounded. They seem friendly and not scared at all. We keep moving towards the largest building to see if we can find their leader and talk to him. I am already thinking what it is we have that might be of value to them.

"Is someone in charge here?"

Wherever I ask the question I am met with blank stares.

"Do they even understand us?"

"It's standard GX Dialect", says Reed finally. I have been watching him out of the corner of my eye as he's been looking at his own information, running scans. I am waiting for something useful from him. "- They should be able to understand us". He says finally.

The children that had surrounded has had communicated in words I didn't understand. But then again children are often taught cultural artefact languages in the hope of keeping traditions alive. As a child I remember being made to speak in Tolarian. My tongue twisting around the phonetic acrobatics it required. Parents continue to visit upon their children whatever hang-ups they might have themselves, perpetuating the suffering of the past well into the future. The thought momentarily makes me smile and then I am jolted back to the present.

"There is a large structure just ahead, behind those trees, says Reed. He is directly reading off whatever map is rolling around inside his head. It should be the center of their government."

He's using the term in its generic form. I wonder what sort
of form leadership takes in this place. Probably oligarchical.
Patriarchal or matriarchal. Some sort of rite of passage
that is the vehicle via which power and the right to lead is
transferred. The thoughts help me structure my approach.
I catch the Regulators exchange a quick glance with each
other.

"Let's go. I say and this time I reach out and grab Sam
and Raynar and push them ahead of me. Sam stumbles
but catches herself, bumps into her partner who grunts in
surprise."

I get the sense they know something I need to know and,
Regulator training manual material, they are withholding it
hoping for an advantage. Something to help them escape.
Reed's map reading takes us outside the village, past thick
trees and along a path we would never have found without
guidance. In a clearing that's evidently maintained at great
physical cost stands a pyramidal structure.

Steps cut into the wood and stone it's made of lead to an
opening at its very top. Talk about a throwback. I have

visions of old Technicolor movies from the 20th century. Ancient explorers coming upon natives hidden deep in Terran jungles. This place is an anachronism in ways that I have never met before.

We make our way up the steps. The Regulators in front of me. Everyone else trailing behind.

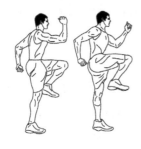
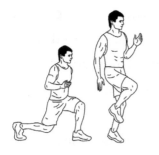

20 march steps

8 lunge step-ups

20 march steps

8 lunge step-ups

20 march steps

8 lunge step-ups

20 march steps

8 lunge step-ups

20 march steps

8 lunge step-ups

There are 357 steps to the top. I count them as I take in
the details around us. The jungle around the structure is
thick, impenetrable almost yet eerily silent. It bugs me.
The number of steps bugs me. I am about to ask Reed to
check for their significance, see if there is something we are
missing here when there is movement at the very top of the
structure and a man emerges.

He's dressed in the same patched up leather as the people we
met at the village behind but he's wearing a necklace made
of stone and in his left hand he's holding a spear. I twitch
a little at the sight of it. The Regulators stop dead in their
tracks. I bring up my hand stopping everyone else behind me
so we don't bump into each other.

"Strangers." The man says.

He's using standard GX Dialect. Part of my brain recalls the
training I've had. Galactic Exchange is a standard language
used across the Terran Universe. It is based upon English
with a simplified, utilitarian structure that takes the romance
out of it. The running joke used to be that it's great for

negotiating a treaty but impossible to use if you're trying to establish a relationship with someone which meant that most probably the all-mighty empire builders rising out of old Terra might have been great diplomats but piss-poor human beings.

"Hi." I say back. "Are you the man in charge?"

"I am Nedlom, son of Meldom and leader of this city."

Okayyy. The village is a 'city' and there is a distinct lack of imagination when it comes to naming children but apart from that everything else is as one would expect in a place like this. The succession line in the name is also an artefact. Without bio IDs how can you establish any kind of credible presence?

"I am Sef, I say. We landed on your planet out of necessity. We need some help."

He lets my words sink in before he nods. Then, with a grand gesture he motions for us to follow him inside.

The inside of the structure is hollow. Huge. Dark. There are torches selectively placed here and there but their light almost doesn't make it to our eyes. There is a large fire pit in the middle of the structure and something suspended above it. Smoke is rising from it. Incense. Great.

There are people gathered around the fire pit. A lot of them. Mostly men but also some women. They are standing still looking up at us as we follow Nedlom down a series of zig-zagging steps that are designed to take us to the bottom of the structure.

It strikes me as odd. We had to ascend, from the outside. Enter at the very top and inside we have to descend, in stages, heading for the bottom.

"Basic religious ritual structure." - Reed says almost reading my thoughts. He's been scanning a database. The ascend from the outside is cleansing. There were 357 steps. "The numbers 3, 5 and 7 come out of old Terra's Egyptian past. They stand for Plurality, Death or Punishment and Perfection or Completeness."

"And the descend?"

"That's unstructured. There is no logic to the number of steps we are going down on and each set stops at a landing that takes us to the beginning of another set of steps. I suspect it's just the descend that matters not the steps."

"Descend into what?"

Sam, the Regulator, turns around, looks at me, almost as if to say something but Raynar throws her a look that stops her. The girl has been walking behind us, bringing up the rear all this time. Now she speaks up.

"This is really primitive. These people still worship some sort of local god."

"What?" I hiss. This is knowledge I can use in my negotiations with their leader.

"The steps, the set up. I-, my father made me study the ancient archives look at cultures from the past. Whenever you have conditions of extreme impoverishment and Patriarchal power structures you get some kind of convergence with superstitious beliefs that consolidate power. It helps that it requires blind obedience because accepting your leader is part of faith."

"Great." I whisper to her.

I realize that despite my extensive capabilities and skillset there are gaps in my knowledge that reflect my very precise role in the shall we say, more civilized part of the universe?

"Nedlom," I say, and the leader halts his descend and turns to look at me.

"Yes?"

"We need to talk. I need to explain the kind of help we need. What we can do for you in return."

"In a minute." He gestures towards the firepit at the bottom of the structure. "We talk there."

He resumes his descend and we follow.

The root of any negotiation is based upon a mutual need. Both parties negotiate because each needs something in return. This makes any kind of talks like this a delicate thing. Give away what you want too quickly and the other party will re-adjust their position to take advantage of you. Fail to understand what is really important to those you negotiate with and you have no read on what they want, which means you are in no position to make a deal of any kind.

This is hard enough when it takes place in your own culture but across different cultures it becomes even more tricky.

We are at the bottom of the structure with Nedlom seated in what looks like a throne made out of animal bones and probably his entire tribe gathered in a tight circle around us.

The talk has been going on for an hour already during which we established that the village has almost everything it needs. Now 'everything' is a matter of perspective. So really I am probing to find what it is we can give them in return for the Xelium we need.

Nedlom, for all his projected majesty is actually not very well versed in the GX Dialect. He uses expressions that are bastardized versions of GX speech and I have to guess at what he really means. When I explain that we have scientific know-how that could materially benefit his village he motions towards someone at the very back of the crowd.

There is movement and a murmur and after some jostling someone is brought forward and thrown on the ground at our feet. It's a woman. Short dark hair. Stout of body. Around middle aged. Dressed in standard Corporate Planetary Explorer uniform although it is now, more than just a little tattered. Her hands are tied behind her back but apart from that she appears to be unharmed.

"What is this?" I ask.

I see the Regulators exchange that glance again and my senses ramp up. It's really hot near the fire pit. The smoke from the fire, the heat it gives off, the stupid incense plus the smells and heat from who knows how many unwashed bodies combines to dull your sense of the surroundings.

"This is Tessa." Says Nedlom. "Our scientist."

She was, it transpires, part of a much larger expeditionary force that came to this planet. It makes sense of course. A Xelium-rich planet cannot long be allowed to plot its own course.

"Where are the others?" I ask.

"Gone." Says Nedlom gesturing towards the space above us with both arms.

The roof of the structure is lost in darkness, high above our heads. I can't even make out the opening we came through. As a matter of fact my eyes can't focus too well. The stupid heat and the smoke are affecting me.

"Gone?" I ask stupidly. Nedlom nods vigorously. Almost with glee. Tessa, on the ground still looks frozen.

"You want fuel". Nedlom says, his eyes shining.

After such long time pussy-footing around everything it's almost a relief.

"Yes", I nod. "We can give you medicine in return. Solar generators for light and heat too." I purposely do not offer weapons. I may not be a student of the Ancient Archives like Ellie but I understand human nature only too well. And I have a conscience, despite what others say about me.

"Medicine." Nedlom repeats the word slowly. Unnecessarily. It's almost like he is playing for time.

"What happened to your crew?" I ask Tessa in Corporate High Language.

"Dead". Is her monosyllabic reply.

Negotiations are a puzzle. You take elements that you possess. Let's call that knowledge. And you add everything that you know. Let's call that memory and then you filter everything through the dynamic of two parties interacting. Circling around something. That is context. Context changes everything.

I see Sam, the Regulator, finally looking straight at me. Her eyes a plea or a warning. Tessa is still on the ground. Hands tied behind her back. Head bowed in submission. The primitive village's tamed scientist.

Ellia and Reed are oddly silent. A little glassy eyed. The heat and the smoke. The incense. The incense! And part of me mines a memory of such a long time ago. The setting white, clinical. A whole line of wire-framed skeletons placed in a row in front of us. I am part of a group. Students learning deadly skills. Expert instructors advising us of the best way to break human bones, apply sudden, explosive pressure that damages the skeleton of another person. The bones are clean, white. High-molded for perfection and modelled precisely on human bone tolerances.

Their contours exact matches for the human counterpart. Their shape and size adjusted for imperfections and dirt. My mind maps, on its own now, the bones of the throne Nedlom is seated on.

At that moment Tessa looks up at me. The incense! What are they putting in the incense? Nedlom smiles at me and nods as if he knows we have reached a critical point in our negotiations. I regulate my breath. Notice the Regulators appear to be doing that also.

The firepit. The cauldron above it. I recognize it now for what it is. I am not yet completely affected by the incense. The Regulators are trained to resist it too, but even they have limits. Ellie and Reed are too far gone I guess. I will need to drag them along. We shall have to grab Tessa too.

"Cannibals". I whisper to no one in particular but Tessa reads my lips. She lets out a small whimper.

From a pocket I take out a small heat charge. It's blaster-based and intended to create a loud disorientating bang. The thing is I cannot use it without affecting us too. All of us.

"On the ship", I say, "we have a problem with noise. Every time the engine overheats there is a whining noise that comes from it. It really hurts our ears. It is almost redzone deafening."

The Regulators perk up. Redzone is the signal for danger alert. They both nod they understand. I have no time to check if everyone else is on board. We may, quite literally, be out of time. I flick my wrist and throw the charge in the fire pit. I squat down and cover my ears with both hands. The Regulators and even Reed do the same. Tessa, can't. Her hands are tied behind her back. She takes a deep, deep breath and tightens her abdominal muscles elevating her internal fluid pressure. It's a good tactic. Not as effective as covering your ears and shutting your eyes but it helps.

Ellie is the only one who doesn't respond. She has no real concept of what is going on.

The heat charge explodes. There is a deafening bang followed by the familiar push of the pressure wave against the skin. To the unprepared it is like a kick has been placed in the center of their body from the inside. Their eyes go momentarily blind as the ultra-white flash of the charge sears their retina, overloads its capacity to deal with light and momentarily depletes the body's capacity for vision. Their ears give in to the pressure wave. The ringing that follows induces vertigo and vomiting. For large crowd incapacitation there is nothing like a heat charge.

I grab Ellie as she's about to faint. I have no desire to lose her at this stage. I mention for Reed to grab Tessa and set her free. The Regulators are already balancing on the balls of their feet, ready for action.

"Run!" I yell.

And we're off and running. Nedlom, blown off his human bones throne is crawling around on his hands and knees in the dark. Helpless as a kitten. Someone, from the very back of the throng where the heat charge would have done the least damage, throws at us a spear. It's guesswork where we are exactly. It misses all of us but finds its mark in someone who's also crawling on hands and knees, striking him in the lower back and pinning him to the floor like a butterfly.

He gives a loud howl and then lies still.

"Run! Run!" I am pointing towards the series of steps leading to the very top of the structure and the steps that are outside.

We shall have to run all the way to our ship. Blaster in hand. Preying I do not have to use it. I watch as everyone starts climbing at top speed. I follow behind. Ellie's dead weight on my shoulder, lungs burning and legs screaming with pain.

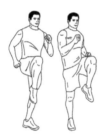

100 high knees

We escape. Barely. Without having to kill anyone. A fluke.

Later, as we are floating through space and in the relative safety of our ship I have time to recount what happened. It was ignorance that blinded us to begin with.

Cannibals are not the kind of thing you expect to meet these days, though the signs should have tipped us off. A mining planet with no miners, off most trade routes and with people living in a time bubble worshipping some kind of local god king.

It's the kind of memory that makes for a great bar story, provided we survive our current predicament and still manage to find a decent bar at some point in the future.

"Why didn't you say anything?" I address the two Regulators.

They don't want to meet my eyes.

"We weren't sure." Sam offers eventually. "There are stories but, you know, they're just stories."

I get that.

"How's Ellie?" I ask Reed.

"She needs a doctor," I nod. One problem at a time. I turn to Tessa. She's been quietly watching us throughout all this.

"Well, what's your story?"

Chapter 16

Space is an empty inhospitable place. It's full of gravity
wells and wormholes, collapsed stars, meteorites, radiation,
energy waves, particle waves, warped areas of Spacetime,
asteroid fields and dark pockets where stranded ships are
doomed to die in. As a matter of fact space is to be avoided at
all costs unless you have a spaceworthy ship and enough fuel
to run it.

Fuel is not just necessary to make the ship travel. Given a
sufficiently high burst of initial thrust most ships will drift in
the right direction at a decent enough speed and a pilot who
understands space can make clever use of gravity wells to

slingshot where he needs to go so he can conserve fuel and cut down his journey time. Fuel is used for other things. It powers the ship's onboard devices. It maintains life support so we can have oxygen to breathe. It runs the generators that spin the hull so we feel that there is gravity on board even when there isn't. It is the life force behind our scanners and weapons systems. And it is what keeps the shields that protect us from the radiation of space, humming quietly.

Fuel, in other words, is what actually keeps humans alive in space. Although we drink water and breathe oxygen we actually run on fuel. Our civilization runs on fuel. Take fuel away from us and we revert to protozoan tethered to a rock and helplessly looking up at the sky.

When I say "fuel" I actually mean Xelium. The great Terran intergalactic empire is a Xelium-based empire. We've all grown up with stories of how Xelium was first discovered deep within the crust of the origin planet. How it changed chemistry forever and made space travel possible. How it was so plentiful once you knew where to look and how to look and how to mine it that it would last us until the heat death of the universe. Xelium is, was and always would be the backbone that made us stand up, gather ourselves and launch our might into the sky.

And now, here, we are running out of Xelium as we burn our way through space. I have a brief image of gold fish being carried in a plastic bag with a tiny hole in it. Their projected lifespan measured by the rate at which the droplets escape through the tiny hole.

We don't have a hole but we can't navigate this ship in any other way apart from burning fuel. None of us is a pilot who's good enough to get through space using all the other smart means of speed augmentation clever pilots know how to use.

It's a predicament that bums me. I have come too far already to turn into a popsicle. My blood boiling in my veins as gravity and hull pressure fail us. My brain dying for lack of oxygen. My body, frozen in space forever. I shake my head to make the image go away. I think wryly to myself that I am making this all about me.

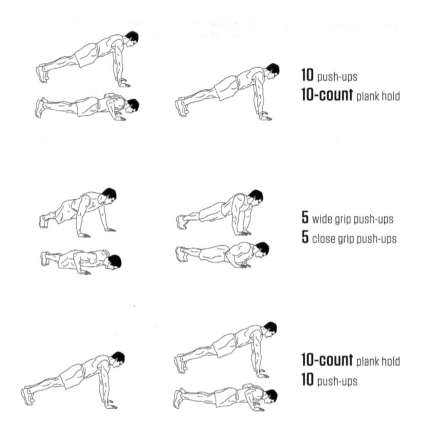

10 push-ups
10-count plank hold

5 wide grip push-ups
5 close grip push-ups

10-count plank hold
10 push-ups

I drop to the floor and do some push ups. I start light and begin to go faster, deeper, changing my grip to work triceps more, then chest, then a wide grip for that extra challenge. Then the plank.

The activity works up a healthy sheen of sweat and clears my head. I think of what Tessa told us.

"I am a doctor," she began. "I was part of a Corp Assignment to help indigenous people on GT-designated planets. Our job was to make sure local populations were fit for mine-duty. We got to the planet surface but something happened to our ship. A week in we lost all contact. Without communications relay we were stranded. Without a mothership we had no eyes on the planet. The tribes people caught us. My comrades ...." she faltered at that point.

Continued: "We ... they took us the same place they took you. We became part of their ritual sacrifice. The feasting afterwards ..." her voice was tight with remembered horror. Her eyes glassy with fear. "They ate them! They ate my crew!"

I asked her how she had been spared. "I'm a doctor. They saw some value in that. Kept me round to tend to their sick. They watched me all the time. If any of their sick should die, they said, that would be it for me. It'd mean my magic had failed and I was now to be shared amongst the tribe like my crew had been. Shared! That's what those savages call eating human flesh!"

There was disgust and horror in equal measure in that voice. I could understand that. I too remembered all too clearly the prickling feeling of icy cold fear at the nape of my neck the moment I realized that we were in a box of sorts, surrounded by people who saw us as lunch.

In getting out of there we'd been lucky. Things could have gone the other way so easily. The thought made me shiver.

The moment I feel locked down by fear I need to do something to help me deal with it. From where I was I asked Reed to run a full area scan and run diagnostics on the ship. I wanted to know which systems we could safely shut down to conserve power and extend our fuel. I then set off to check on the Regulators.

Sam and Raynar were back in their cells. Angry glares on their faces.

"You're back!" Sam spoke up first. "How about letting us out of here? We can help and keeping us locked up when we all are going to die is not clever."

"I'll be the judge of that," I said softly, my eyes taking in Raynar. The bruise on his face where I'd hit him last was fading. It somehow made him look even angrier. "How about you big man?" I say to him, "Do you want to help also?"

He lets a sneer cross his face. "You took me by surprise last time. It won't happen again."

"You will refuse to be surprised?"

"You know what I mean. You got in a lucky punch is all."

Maybe it's the way he said it, or maybe in all this tension and the impending feel of doom and helplessness this became just the release I feel I need. I use the control on my wrist to drop the field generator on their cell just long enough to enter. Lock it up behind me.

"I am here now." I say and with a low growl he lunges at me.

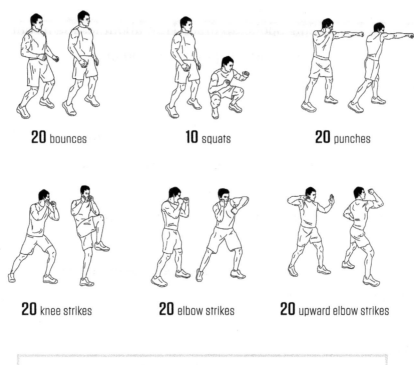

20 bounces   **10** squats   **20** punches

20 knee strikes   **20** elbow strikes   **20** upward elbow strikes

catch your breath, rest up to 2 minutes, and repeat the circuit
7 times in total

Fighting in a closed space takes a special kind of skill. You
have to be aware of every tiny inch around you. How the
walls and furniture eat into your floor space. Where the
corners are in relation to where you're standing. How your
reach versus your opponent's. It's rhythmic ballet merged
into a puzzle, merged into a battle. You're solving for
space and motion even as you're probing for strengths and
weaknesses. Raynar was Regulator-trained. Fast and strong.

But speed and strength are only one component here. Spatial awareness and puzzle solving are also key. As is the ability to sense the rhythm of your opponent's movements.

I fully expected Sam to join in. I was prepared to take on both. She didn't move a muscle. And after a minute or so of my elbows and knees doing damage Raynar was ready to concede defeat.

"You didn't let us die back there with the Cannibals," Sam said eventually. She was darting her eyes from me to Raynar, lying on the floor groaning and wiping blood off his face.

"I am not a monster. I do only what I have to." I don't really need to explain myself to her of all people.

"If we promise to not cause trouble. Really. Will you let us help? Raynar doesn't mean to be an ass. He's just mad you beat him so easily the first time. Now I think he's beginning to get it was no fluke." Her voice, as she says this, is pointed. Raynar groans some more but props himself on one elbow on the floor. His face ain't pretty.

"You did not get lucky," he says finally. "Sam is right. You need our help and we need yours to get out of this. We get to civilized space we'll hitch a ride to our base. You can just take off."

I look at them both and the exchange is real enough to make us all realize that we have no choice. If we don't work together we may not make it at all.

"OK," I concede dropping the field generator and leaving the cell open. "I will explain this to the rest. At the first sign of trouble -"

"There won't be any. Really." Sam cuts me off. She looks at Raynar. He nods quickly and puts out a hand stained with his own blood.

"Shake?"

I take it.

The ship's comms beep once and then Reed's voice comes through: "Sef, we need you in sick bay."

I turn to the two Regulators. "Get to the bridge," I say, "See what you can do to help improve fuel efficiency." I turn and run to the sick bay.

Ellie is strapped on a medbed with probes active around her. Tessa has her back to the door, her eyes glued on the monitor readings.

"How is she?"

She turns at my entrance, eyeing me up. "Not that well," she says. "I've been scanning her for concussion but her neurals are normal. Her vitals also read normal."

"Then?"

"It's her brain waves. She's in Theta. Deep Theta. It's like whatever was in that incense we were breathing down there affected her the most.

"And?"

"I don't know. This ship doesn't come equipped with neural neutralizers or a deep diagnostics med lab. I am doing what I can with what I have. I have her brain mildly sedated to allow cross-messaging across associative neural centers. It will seek to reach homeostasis on its own. Balance its processing by making sense of input. That should help snap her out of it."

"Should?"

She shrugs her shoulders in a most undoctor-like way. "It's the best I can do with what I have here," she motions at the ship's primitive sick bay.

"OK," I feel frustrated, helpless. Angry. I fight down the red tide rising inside me. Turn to leave. "See what you can do to help her," I say unnecessarily. The ship's comms interrupts me again.

"Sef?" It's Reed's voice. "You'd better get to the bridge, we have company."

I start running to get there as fast as possible, wondering what gods I've pissed on in my life and why are they now pissing back on me.

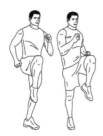

100 high knees

"What is it Reed?" I gasp as I am running, out of breath already. I wonder if the life support systems of the ship have started to slow down. Is its atmosphere thinner? I shouldn't be out of breath so fast.

"A ship. You asked me to scan the area. We're picking up a ship approaching us." Reed's voice sounds preternaturally calm. I have learnt to read people. Understand how they function under pressure. So far Reed has been a really cool customer. He focuses on the things he understands and uses his own enhanced body to work out solutions.

He filters out everything else. Things he cannot control he simply tunes out. It's a remarkable capacity born out of his work in systems that run on pure code. The calmness I sense however is odd. Even for him.

"What's going on?"

"You'll see."

I get to the bridge seriously out of breath. Sam and Raynar are both there, bent over instrumentation, looking at the telemetrics coming in.

"This doesn't make sense," Raynar finally murmurs.

"What's going on?" I ask again.

"The ship Reed spotted," Sam is the first to reply. "It's one of ours. No doubt about it. But it failed to respond to all of our hails."

"Is it getting ready to attack?" I ask, "Are its weapons systems going hot?"

"No, that's just it." Reed finally says. His voice is perplexed. "I've run deep scans inside it. It's moving our way but there are no signs of life."

"What?"

"Reed thinks it's drifting," Sam adds. "It's a ghost ship."

Chapter 17

"The scans are still coming back empty," Reed says. "No sign of life. I am sure."

The two Regulators, busy at their screens, confirm this curtly. I notice they don't talk much and I kinda like that. I haven't had time to explain their presence to the others on the Bridge but judging by the fact that they are at instrument consoles, they must have explained it themselves.

I see Reed doing something strange with his eyes and it dawns on me just how long he's been deep in whatever machine code interface he goes into every time he plugs in.

The eyes are the one part of us that get tired regardless. Like any hacker whose body has been instrumentalized Reed has developed personal strategies to help him get past fatigue and the lack of focus that comes with routine work. The eye exercises he is doing are energizing as well as a natural de-stresser for the eyes.

"Keep scanning for movement," I say to the two Regulators. "Anything moves on that dead ship I want to know."

They look a little surprised but they are professional. Once freed from the cell and their collars they don't feel the need to challenge anyone's authority. Plus, they know my command makes sense. There may be no overt signs of life on that Ghost Ship but the legends around them didn't materialize out of thin air.

Space is awash with energies. Energy and matter are interchangeable. For most of us that is only of academic interest. The frequency boundaries that help us maintain our carbon-based cellular form are not quite so accommodating when ships jump in and out of near light speeds, next to deep gravity wells, awash with exotic energies. No one quite knows how Ghost Ships come about but one theory has it that the humans within are transformed; their matter turned into energy, their corporeal coherence ruptured for good.

The most famous Ghost Ship was the Saratoga. The jewel of the origin planet's magnificent battle wagons. Large as a moon. Sleek as a space needle. Armed with enough weaponry to put a few black holes in your average galactic cluster. When it disappeared everyone thought it'd simply gone to ground, it was after all at the height of the Corporation Wars. It was decades before it came back, floating serenely through Terran space. All systems dark. When it was boarded nothing was found. The ship itself was intact. Meals in the gulley abandoned half-eaten like crew members had somehow dematerialized in mid-meal. No signs of battle or damage anywhere. But no sign of the crew either.

It's not like an entire crew, almost 1,000 men and women, can go missing in the middle of a patrol. When the Saratoga's records were examined they showed that the ship had set out on a routine patrol mission beyond Mars. Shortly after orbiting the Red Planet it had gone dark.

Scientists swarmed over it for months. Tests were carried
out. Nothing.

And then the tales started to fly about. Told in hushed tones
from outpost to outpost. Rumors of strange reflections
in mirrors aboard the ship. Motion sensors picking up
movement when there was nothing to see. Those who had
been studying it started to have hallucinations. Some went
mad and took their own lives. Others disappeared. Just got
up and left one night, never to be seen again.

Energy is not always strictly compartmentalized. I know
that well. Maybe all this is just the stories put out by minds
strained by work exhaustion or boredom or fear. The brain
latching onto likely explanations for unlikely events, however
superstitious they may seem. The fact is Ghost Ships are
given a wide berth. Everyone's lives are tangled up enough
without additional complications. Unless there is no other
choice.

We were out of other choices.

"I have motion!" from Raynar.

"Me too!" Confirmed Sam, a second later.

Great! Their voices sent Reed scuttling out of his eye exercises and back on his scans.

"No heat signature," he says. "Strange. And no life signs either."

Yet something had moved. The Regulators' scanners had picked up movement.

"Get the doctor up here," I say to Sam, "she's in sick bay." I watch her move fast, with confidence, as she makes her way to get Tessa. "We need the fuel that ship is carrying," I say to no one in particular and catch the tiny twitch from Raynar, before he controls it. He's heard the Ghost Ship rumors too, then.

"You think it's worth the risk?" He asks.

I shrug my answer. Then: "What choice do we have?"

It takes us a few hours to get to within visual of the Ghost Ship, put a plan of action together and decide exactly who is going to be involved in its execution. There is much talk and finally we settle on me, Tessa, Sam and Raynar to go in. Reed will stay with Ellie.

Regulator ships are not easy to board, nor do they readily give up their fuel. I know I need Sam and Raynar to help me locate viable fuel cells and extract them. I will need their expertise to dismantle whatever defenses the ship has in place. Tessa in the meantime will scour sick bay. Look for anything she can use to help her treat Ellie. There is guilt tagging at me deep inside here.

Ellie might be the way she is because of me. Maybe the concussion was way stronger than anything I'd anticipated in her case. Maybe the combination of my explosive charge and the incense were enough to damage her brain. Maybe. I wasn't sure why I cared so much really. I barely knew the kid, yet here I was, worrying that I might be the reason she never wakes up from whatever coma she's in, right now.

I wonder, at times, whether the past is catching up with me. Red dust colors my nightmares. I, more than most people, know that we have two lives. One we present to the outside world. That's a normalized one. It's where we, mostly, are what others expect us to be. Do what is expected of us. The other life, the one deep inside us however, we rarely acknowledge. It's the one where we become our own masters. Do what we want. Disregard norms and protocols and pull the trigger turning those who cross our path into piles of red dust.

These two lives are always at war inside us. Which one eventually wins determines the person we become. I shake my head, suddenly conscious the others are looking at me.

"You're not saying anything," Tessa breaks the silence.

"Sorry, I was calculating the odds,"

"On the Ghost Ship?" from Raynar.

I nod. No one says anything else. We all know our roles.

***

Suited up and breathing bottled oxygen reminds me why I hate suiting up and breathing bottled oxygen. It's not just the claustrophobia, the sense that everything is closing in on you. It is the fragility. Suddenly you realize that without special suits, pumps, atmosphere to take with you, your flesh and blood body is just so much useless, organic matter in space.

Reed, I am thinking, would sympathize. Hackers are notoriously intolerant to any weakness of the flesh.

"Sef, keep breathing. Your vitals are dropping." Reed's voice in my ear makes everything real. I take a deep breath and move on. I motion for the others to follow me.

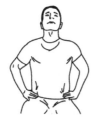

take 3 deep breaths

"Once inside we'll double-check the atmosphere," I say, "if it's OK we use the ship's. Save on our own tanks."

They all nod their agreement. The shuttle that took us across the two ships is tiny by comparison. The Ghost Ship is massive. An armed transporter by the looks of it. Regulator issue, Corps-backed.

"Once inside we split up." I say. I catch Raynar's snort in my ear. I know what he's thinking. Every audiovisual entertainment disaster starts with our heroes splitting up.

"No choice, remember?" I look Raynar's way as I say this for the benefit of everyone. "I want a quick in and out. We're not staying here longer than we need to."

With Reed's help we are able to get past the airlock doors fast. Then, as they close in behind us and ship schematics load up on the display of our helmets, I urge everyone to move fast. We have less than an hour to get everything done.

We all cast one last look at each other. With helmets pushed back, breathing ship oxygen; in the light cast by the ship's emergency lights we all look a little strange. Our irises are too dark and there are dark shadows beneath each eye. It makes us all look a little bit like the dead, already.

Sam and Raynar will look for the fuel cells we need. Tessa has to get to sick bay. I will scout around, see if there is anything else we can use.

"Go," I say, "Go!"

The ship's emergency lights don't function everywhere. Parts of it are either dimly lit or dark. It's cold inside. As I breathe out I can see the cold stream of my breath. While its atmosphere is holding the rest of it is far from hospitable. At the back of my mind I start to wonder just how long it's been drifting like this and I have to forcibly quell the thought and shove what I know about Ghost Ships aside.

With my helmet off I don't have ready access to the visual
schematics Reed loaded for us but I remember the rough
layout of the ship. I find a shaft and descend one deck.

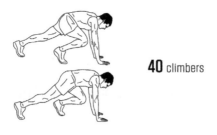

40 climbers

The corridor I find myself in leads to an array of airlocks.
Escape pods lie in wait. Unused. I can see why.

The corridor is littered with bodies. Or rather, body parts.
In the ship's low gravity and cold, blood has coagulated
fast and frozen into globules. The spatter patterns tell
me that something run through this way moving fast. It
dismembered everything in its path. How? What? These are
questions I need to answer but don't just yet know how.
I examine a couple of bodies and they are in a terrible state.

Their wounds are consistent with blunt force trauma. If they'd been run over by a fast truck I would have understood but here, in space. As a precaution I unclip my blaster, make sure it's ready to discharge. There must be at least twenty bodies here. They were running, trying to make their way into the pods when whatever was chasing them caught up with them.

I wonder why they're not armed. Why they have no suits on. I know the pods have their own life support but still, standard space protocol says you suit up in a life pod. An added precaution against the kind of glitches that leak your atmosphere out into space and end your timeline sooner than it should end.

They were caught by surprise is the natural assumption of course. Again, how? By what? Questions, questions. There is nothing in what I see to give me a clue. No claw marks. No energy burns.

"Sef, we've found the fuel cells," Raynar's voice interrupts me.

"I've found the crew," I answer back. "What's left of them. Stay sharp."

"Affirmative." The Regulator falls back into standard battle talk.

I remember the sick bay is a level below me still. I look for an airlock to take me there. My guess is where Tessa is and I need to round her up and get back to the Regulators. The first airlock I try is stuck fast. It won't budge no matter what I try. I find a service tunnel and squeeze through the opening panel, I start to climb down.

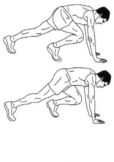
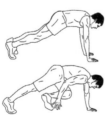

20 climbers

2 climber taps

20 climbers

2 climber taps

20 climbers

2 climber taps

20 climbers

2 climber taps

20 climbers

2 climber taps

The sick bay, when I get to it is empty. No sign of Tessa. There is more blood though. A lot of blood. Blood spatter just like in the corridor above. It spells bad news for whoever had been here when whatever happened had happened.

The place gives me the creeps and the creeps is something I listen to. The subconscious signals that read danger are processed by the mind at levels well beneath conscious awareness. Listening to them, when they surface, requires a special kind of awareness. My subconscious has kept me alive more times than my conscious. I am not about to start ignoring its warnings.

I have the blaster out now. I inch away from the empty sick bay. The corridor is dimly lit. There are dark patches ahead. When I squint I can see body parts. Worse than above. I move slowly forward all senses on the alert.

There are several chambers leading off it. Through their glass panels I can see equipment in some sort of disarray. Gurneys. It looks like medical labs. I recall nothing on the ship's manifest about this. There is the low sound of metal scraping on metal from somewhere ahead and I feel my blood freeze.

My steps become silent as my body tenses for action. I am sure there is someone there with me. In one of the chambers ahead. I inch my way along the wall, eyes checking everything carefully. I dry swallow to clear the constriction on my throat. My pulse is attempting to race but I quickly bring it under control.

I edge up to the door of the next chamber. Peer inside through the panel. The panel is smeared with blood from the inside, making it hard to see everything. There is movement. There is the same sound of metal scraping on metal as someone tries to push a large metal cabinet away from a workstation where it has been crashed against.

Before I can think consciously I am inside the chamber. Blaster raised. Then:

"Tessa."

She spins around in shock. Loses her balance as she does so, clearly startled, begins to fall. I am quick enough to catch her before she hits the floor.

"You scared me!" she gasps.

"Did you find medical supplies?" I look behind her at the complex array of medical equipment and medscan devices on the workstation. The cabinet she'd been trying to move was blocking access to most of them.

"Not in sick bay. There's the equipment I need right there," she points to the workstation.

I help her slide the heavy metal cabinet away from the workstation and she quickly picks out some of the equipment she needs and several unlabeled boxes of medicine.

"What is this place?" I ask her.

There's no answer and I am not even sure she's heard me. I look about the empty gurneys. They all have heavy, leather restraints and all of them are covered in blood. Whoever was in them clearly did not have a good time.

"It's not even in the schematics," I say, mostly to myself. I watch Tessa expertly navigate her way round the room, skirting the bloodied gurneys with ease, opening drawers from the wall behind them, taking out specific medicine boxes and specialized syringes and other equipment.

"Good to go," she says at last.

Not a moment too soon.

"Sef? We need some muscle here," from Raynar.

"We're on our way," I motion to Tessa and blaster in hand I bring up the rear as she unerringly picks her way back to where Raynar and Sam are struggling with a fuel cell.

My senses are still on alert. My gut feeling to danger has not gone away. Without a specific cause of danger to absorb my attention I am in real danger of overloading. My brain shutting down. It's that bad. The task of extracting the fuel cell is a welcome distraction.

"Everything OK?" Raynar notices the blaster I am still holding. I nod as I holster it at my side.

"Let's get to work," I say.

Ununoctium is the heaviest element in the universe. To understand fuel cell technology you need to consider that Xelium, the substance that can be mined virtually everywhere, when mixed with Ununoctium, in a specialized reactor, generates force equivalent to several million times its volume while oxidizing at the same rapid reaction rate as the old aluminum-based, solid-fuel compounds of the old Terra technology.

For those who did not pay attention in their intergalactic history class this means that a mix of Ununoctium and Xelium are about as close as rocket fuel technology will ever get to a "free lunch". A small amount goes a long way and part of the byproducts produced kick off a replenishing cycle now known as the Carbide Trade-Off, named after a defunct Terran Corporation, that reconstitutes a certain percentage of the original mass.

All that makes fuel cells very compact and very, very heavy.
Raynar and I braced and lifted. The fuel cell was balanced
on rods that made it easier to move but overcoming inertia
was not easy. I could feel my muscles bulge and groan under
my suit as I strained against the load. Raynar was breathing
heavily and grunting.

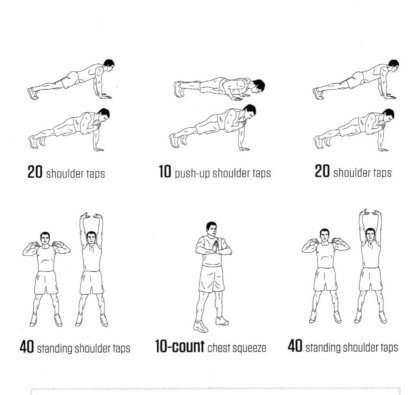

20 shoulder taps   **10** push-up shoulder taps   **20** shoulder taps

40 standing shoulder taps   **10-count** chest squeeze   **40** standing shoulder taps

catch your breath, rest up to 2 minutes, and repeat the circuit
7 times in total

"Let me help," Sam pitted her own strength against the impossibly heavy metal.

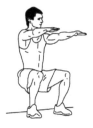

60 Seconds wall sit

For a long minute nothing moved. It appeared almost as if we wouldn't be enough. At the very last moment, when I was about to swear loudly and stop pulling against the load of the fuel cell, something popped, deep somewhere in the machinery. The fuel cell moved. A tiny fraction.

"It's moving!" Raynar said through gritted teeth.

I nodded and redoubled my efforts. Sam strained. Tessa, arms full of the equipment and supplies she'd salvaged, watched. Another give. Then another. With the groan of metal being moved after a long time, the fuel cell rose majestically from its berthing.

We now pushed instead of pulling as the heavy cylinder rose above us, its base still in its berth.

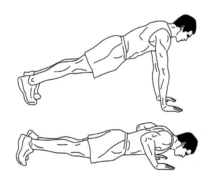

10 push-ups

catch your breath

10 push-ups

catch your breath

10 push-ups

catch your breath

10 push-ups

catch your breath

10 push-ups

"You've got a transporter?" Raynar gasped at me, sweat sliding down his face from the effort.

I couldn't answer back. My face was equally drenched with sweat. I pointed with my eyes. Just a step or two behind me was the circular, wheeled base designed to take the exact shape and weight of a fuel cell. Once locked in it a baby could push it around.

"Ok, then," from Raynar.

"On my count," I gasped, "One, two, three!" We all heaved. The fuel cell came out with a final wrench and we just managed to maneuver it to its transporter wheel base. "Phew!" from Sam.

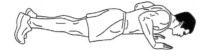 **30 Seconds** push-up plank hold

I began to smile when Tessa who had been watching us silently let out a warning cry: "Look out! It's a Chimera!"

A shadow detached itself from the far end of the room and sprang off the floor with a mighty leap. It bounced off the wall, blunt face forward. Beady, dark eyes, designed to catch more of the light spectrum than human eyes ever could.

Chimeras were illegal. Artificially spliced organisms made from a concoction of human and animal DNA. They were used as bioweapons in the first Corporate war against the Apostates from Terra. Bred to kill they would wipe out entire divisions. Supernaturally fast, fearless. Resistant to pain, cold, heat, hunger and thirst, they'd been outlawed.

Its presence here explained a lot about what had happened on this Ghost Ship and its crew. However it had got aboard, the creature could take on any number of armed men and, given time, dismantle an entire ship. Engineered to survive deep space legend had it they were immortal. Capable of using solar radiation to maintain vital signs until they could get aboard a ship or find a planet.

And now we had to deal with one. This trip just kept getting better and better.

If Raynar immediately recognized the level of the threat or not is immaterial. On Tessa's shouted warning he acted with Regulator-honed reaction. He flung himself away from the fuel cell, shoulder-rolled on the floor ducking what would have been a decapitating blow from the creature and springing to his feet, just behind it.

It was a clever move. Not enough. Chimera's, for all their brute power, were intelligent. Human DNA made them adaptive and adaptable. The creature let out a blood-curdling scream of rage at having missed its target. Arresting its momentum it stopped and kicked back, where Raynar was springing to his feet. The move caught the Regulator by surprise. A half step forward on his part and his rib cage would have been splintered, his lungs collapsed. Heart probably destroyed.

He was lucky in springing up just out of reach. By the time the kick hit him, he'd reflexively crossed his arms in front of him absorbing some of the momentum and had began to backpedal. The kick pushed him with force so that he crashed against the metal bulkhead behind him but he was alive and relatively unhurt. His arms, numb from absorbing the power of the blow, were temporarily useless to him.

The Chimera turned and lunged for him. That was a mistake. I don't know exactly what team spirit existed with the Regulators on the ship but here no one turned and ran when the others were in trouble. Focusing on killing Raynar the Chimera ignored me.

It takes less than a second for a blaster to be unholstered, aimed and fired and in that time the Chimera had crossed the space between it and Raynar, had grabbed him with a powerful hand from the front of his suit and was busy raising its fist, taking the time to aim at his head, intent on obliterating him completely.

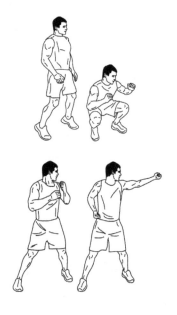

2 squats

20 backfists, right arm

hop and change sides

2 squats

20 backfists, left arm

hop and change sides

2 squats

20 backfists, right arm

hop and change sides

2 squats

20 backfists, left arm

The high-pitched voice of the blaster came in the instant between the creature raising its fist and launching its punch. It caught it with its fist less than a hand's width from impact with Raynar's unprotected head. The exotic energies of the blaster worked on it the same way they work on human flesh. They dissolved the molecular boundaries that keep an organic form together at a cellular level. They evaporated all liquids contained within its shape. They then found the heavier elements in its bones and dissolved the matrix that kept them together, releasing a small flash of energy. They then burned all minerals away in an exogenic reaction that turns an organism into a pile of red dust. They did all this in microseconds. The Chimera seemed to vanish in a puff of mist from evaporated liquids and light from burning minerals. A few grains of red dust danced in the air where it had been. A small pile of them was at Raynar's feet.

"Thanks," Raynar turned to me, rubbing feeling back into his arms.

"Let's get the fuel cell back to the ship. This place is a graveyard for a reason." I say and motion for everyone to get to work.

Chapter 18

After the Ghost Ship, our own ship seemed like the safest

space in the world. You need to understand something about

danger and safety. It is always relative. If I throw you in the

middle of a war zone and I've plucked you out of a birthday

party, you'll freeze. Your muscles will go on lockdown. Your

heart rate will spike. Your lungs will seize up as you gasp for

breath and your adrenaline levels will go through the roof.

The most spectacular change however will be invisible. If

you could see your brain under these conditions you will see

a dozen neural centers all lit up like Christmas trees, firing

off messages that will fail to get where they're supposed to because your brain will be awash with cortisol, the stress hormone. Cortisol shuts down some of the higher centers of the brain which means the messages you most need in order to survive are simply not getting through. The overload in chemicals that zip about but achieve nothing soon creates its own gridlock. Your survival is totally not guaranteed.

I have been in war zones. The reason my brain doesn't shut down like that is the same as the Regulators. We've been trained. "Battle hardening" is what they call it in the militarized planets where the War Academies are. Basically they train us to know what to expect. They then train us to expect the unexpected. They teach our brains when to peak and when to chill. We learn to take the relative for what it is and make the most of it. This replenishes the brain's and body's biochemistry and resets us fast.

On board the ship I take a few moments to change the charge on my blaster to a full pack. I then sit in one of the deck seats and just breathe in and out for a few. I feel my lungs open up, my brain come down to normal. Within minutes I am good to go again.

Out of the corner of my eye I see Raynar do the same. He's
in a seat. Taking a few deep breaths. Trained professionals
make the most of the downtime they get. There's never
knowing when it will come round again. He takes a little
longer than me to come out of it. It was a close call he
had back there on the Ghost Ship. Close calls take a toll.
Professionals appear to brush them off, take things in their
stride but that's not how it works.

Pain, fear, uncertainty they all build up. Everyone made of
flesh and blood, carbon and dust, responds the same way.
Professionals acknowledge their feelings. They take the
build up and push it away, in a very special place at the very
back of their mind. And from there, they will pull it back to
the front and examine it again, at some other time, when it
will be safe to do so. When the heart palpitations and hand
tremors and eye twitches will not be incapacitating because
there will be no danger around. That's how professionals
deal with this.

"Good to go?" I ask Raynar. He nods. Peels himself off the
seat he'd been in. Checks to see if I am still armed. It's a
subconscious thing. "Reed's off to do his thing with the
power cell-"

I am cut off by a scream. It comes through the intercom loud and clear. There is real pain in it. Agonizing pain. The sort of thing that cannot be faked. And it's Sam's.

"Where?" Raynar begins.

"Level below," I say. My eyes are already scanning the monitors to see if there are any active feeds. I don't see anything we can use so we both break into a sprint to get there fast.

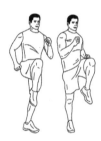

200 high knees

We hit the corridor at a breakneck pace. There is one more agonizing scream over the intercom and it's cut short.
The silence makes our hearts pound harder. Raynar and I clamp down on the fear. Our legs work and our arms pump and we reach the shaft that will take us to the level below simultaneously.

I dive in first. I'm known for my impulsiveness in the face
of the unknown. Or at least that's what I've heard. Raynar is
hard on my heels.

I hit the deck, blaster in hand and eyes scanning the space.
It's a holding area. Empty. The kind that ships have that
doubles as anything they need it to be. Empty space is easy to
convert. What was Sam doing here? Where-

I see the blood. There is a lot of it. A long, thick trail that
ends up in a pool by the far side of the hull. The blaster is
poised in front of me now.

"What the-" Raynar gasps and his eyes and mine together
make contact with Sam's body. What's left of it. One of her
arms has been torn off completely. Her body lies at an angle.
Flung like a rag doll. A broken toy. Both legs are folded
under her at the knee. Her chest looks crumpled inside her
Regulator uniform. Ribcage smashed.

I spin around, eyes darting everywhere. It's instinct more
than anything else. I know of only one thing that can do that
kind of damage to a human body. I saw it on the Ghost Ship.
There is movement at the far end. Shadows moving.

At the shaft we dropped down on. I raise the blaster but the movement before I can take any action.

"Chimera," I say. I am not 100% sure, but it looks that way.

"How?" Raynar sounds cool and collected as he runs beside me. Whatever he's feeling he has a tight lid on it.

"I don't know yet. But we need to get it." I liked Sam. From the two Regulators she had definitely been the one with the better sense of self control and better brains.

"Yes," Raynar's tense.

"Reed," I say on the comms. "Can you hear me?"

"What's up?"

"What's the situation with the fuel cell?"

"I have everything in place. I am running diagnostics but it all looks good so far. We should be able to get going in maybe 40 minutes."

"Ok. Listen. We have a Chimera on board."

"What?" Reed's voice, usually so cool, loses some of its customary coolness.

"Get everyone on the bridge."

"Everyone?" he asks.

"Yes. Especially Tessa and the girl. Sick bay is way too accessible." Sick bays by their very nature are.

"OK."

"Button down the bridge. Get us underway. Let no one else in apart from me and Raynar." It's a second or two before it sinks in. He's running scans maybe to confirm.

Then: "What about Sam. The Regulator?"

"She's dead." I have a terrible way of breaking bad news, I know. "This thing killed her. Raynar and I are going to get it. Out."

"You'd better have this," I say to Raynar. In my hand I am holding a second blaster. A little less powerful than the one at my waist. A back-up piece for me. Just as lethal. Just as accurate.

He takes it without a word. Getting Sam's killer and making sure the ship is safe is our priority right now.

Ships are metal cans. With tubes and boxes inside. The tubes get you to the boxes. I know, I know. Shipwrights, the AI-augmented geniuses who build these things would want me tied up and shot if they could hear my description. First, they'd have to take a number and join the queue for that. Second, they can't hear me.

Raynar and I get real busy running, sliding and jumping from tube to box to tube to box again. We try to secure each one by locking the airlocks and sealing the doors but we are just not sure if the Chimera would be able to open them, just like we can. There's just not enough known about these deadly things, except perhaps the fact that they're deadly.

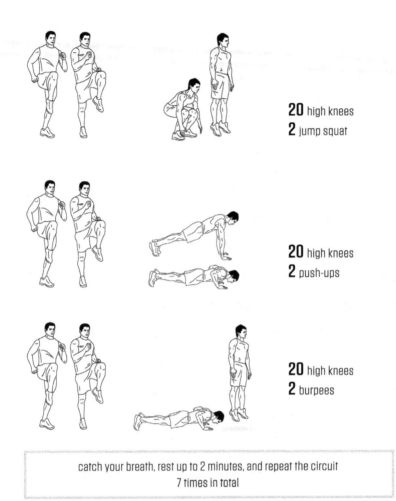

20 high knees
2 jump squat

20 high knees
2 push-ups

20 high knees
2 burpees

catch your breath, rest up to 2 minutes, and repeat the circuit
7 times in total

Hunting a deadly enemy on a ship, in space is a game of narrowing statistics. The more tubes we travel through and the more boxes we secure the higher are the odds that we shall find our quarry. Which means it also stands a higher chance than average of finding us.

"This shit is hard," I am out of breath and sweating heavily. Raynar grants his agreement. He too is covered in sweat.

"Reed," I speak into the comms.

"What?"

"Is the bridge secure?"

"Tightly locked up," Reed confirms. "Just me the doc and the girl here," he says. "By the way, she's awake."

"What?"

"And asking for you,"

I don't have time to deal with this right now. I grant my acknowledgement to Reed and kill the channel.

"Three more compartments to go," Raynar says. "This thing can't double back, right?"

"Nothing's certain but I think it can't."

"Great. I like your certainty."

"An asset under pressure,"

We both smile and it takes the edge off the tension we feel.

"Where did you learn to fight like you do?"

"I grew up rough. Backwater planets are not known for their civility."

Raynar nods at that. "Me too," he says eventually. "I joined the Regulators to get away from Oxygen gangs."

Oxygen gangs! I'd heard the rumors. On small planetary establishments, where the Terraforming process had not yet completed but the immigration had already started, those unlucky enough to have to go first because they had no other choice, sometimes had to fight for air. Oxygen, the most basic commodity needed for human life became a bargaining chip over which lives were enslaved and fortunes lost and made.

Raynar must have grown up on a mining planet then. Like
me. Lives diverge but there are only so many origin stories.
Those born with a silver spoon in our mouth rarely find
themselves in a narrative like mine. Hunting around, blaster
in hand, looking for Chimera that might end me. Inwardly I
sigh.

"Stay sharp," I whisper unnecessarily. I can see from the way
Raynar moves that he is ready for action.

"Roger that," he falls back to his military responses. Talk
helps take the edge off our nervousness. A clink in the deep
shadows to our right has both of us moving as one. We
separate. Both execute picture-perfect shoulder rolls. We
come up, one knee on the floor. Blasters extended. It's a
classic military maneuver: separate to present two targets.

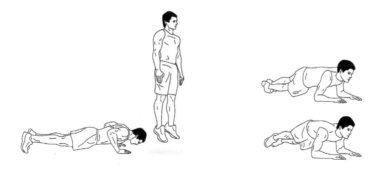

ONE burpee and then 30 plank rolls

Present to the enemy two sources of fire.

You need a good core for moves like that.

There is nothing to see where the sound came from. Damn. "Anything?" Raynar asks quietly. He's scanning the half of the room I am not.

"Nope," I say and we get hit.

The Chimera moves fluidly fast. Its bulk is powered by such strength it moves as if it's weightless, the ship's artificial gravity barely registering. My brain does something weird, it begins to think about gravity wells and how gravity waves are necessary to maintain bone density. It's a response to overwhelming fear. I snap it back to the present. Duck under the Chimera's massive swing. Kick out as I fall back.

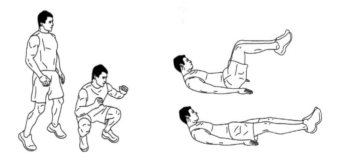

30 squats and then **30** crunch kicks

Both boots make contact. The Chimera's skin feels like concrete. I am flung back. The creature is off by a fraction. My kicks have surprised it. Its miscalculation saves Raynar's life. The Regulator rolls away, fires one blind burst from the blaster. It misses, but the creature flinches. Pauses for a split second. A split second is all I need.

It all happens so fast that my brain sees it in slow mo. The creature rolling in mid-air, twisting round to bring its bulk to bear on us again. Raynar, struggling to regain his balance.

Me, on my back, sliding away from the Chimera and Raynar. Blaster rising slowly. The action in front of me perfectly framed.

There is a burst of light from my right hand. The walls of the hull are briefly lit up by garish silhouettes engaged in some kind of macabre dance. Then there is an unearthly sound and the usual flash of light as the blaster's energies do their job. Red dust molecules hang in midair; twirling slowly as they fall to the cold metal floor.

"Close one," Raynar says noncommittally and I nod.

I begin to rise to my feet. He is already up and holstering his blaster. I notice he's not thinking of giving it up. My brain is working with the blast's after image still fresh on my retinas.

Shadows thrown up on the hull wall. The blaster throwing out outlines. Monstrously exaggerated forms. Raynar, caught on his side, desperately trying to rise looking like some wounded beast with an arched back and horns. The Chimera, framed centre. A massive bulk of black about to be extinguished. The half part of me picked up by the blaster's light falling back into the shadows.

The Shadows! My brain works overtime trying to warn me. I am still fresh with relief. Giddy with our easy victory over the monster that had destroyed the Ghost Ship. And the tableau from that ship rolls unbidden in my mind. Broken bodies jumbled together. Piled in the middle of an airlock. In the middle! Shadows. Dark mass behind me.

Why would bodies be piled up in the middle?

"There's another one-" I begin to cry out and start to twist at the same time.

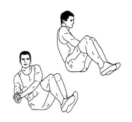

40 sitting twists in one go

Too late. The deep dark shadow behind me materialises into Chimera solidity. My movement, fast as it is, is too slow to save me. "Raynar!"

The blow, when it comes, clips me on left side. I feel more than hear the splintering of bone. The numbness of massive damage. I try to say something more but there is no sound I can hear nor do I have a sense of control over my mouth anymore. I try to fall so that the blaster I am holding is side up, unblocked by the damaged mass of my body, but there is no sense of control in my movements. It's like I have been blown into a massive, invisible, galactic particle stream.

I vaguely have a sense of the metal floor as I hit it. I try as hard as I can to force my finger to squeeze the blaster trigger. My head must hit the floor hard but I only know that because I have a sensation of it bouncing off the floor.

My vision begins to fade and I have a sense of bright beams above me. Raynar's blaster. Still going off?

Is he alive? The Chimera towers over me. So fast. So powerful.

Voices. Screams? I ... fade.

Darkness swallows me.

Chapter 19

Blasts whiz by. Flashes of white that can turn you into red
dust. My lungs gasp for breath. The kid is already heavy in
my arms. My head hurts and I have to blink my eyes rapidly
to clear them of particulates. Red dust permeates the air.

"Hang on kid," I murmur reassuringly and my voice calms
him down. He stops struggling and clings tightly to me. Arms
wrapped round my neck. Head bobbing next to mine as I
pump my knees and make for the cluster of buildings ahead.

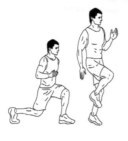
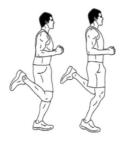

10 lunge step-ups

20 butt kicks

10 lunge step-ups

20 butt kicks

10 lunge step-ups

20 butt kicks

10 lunge step-ups

20 butt kicks

10 lunge step-ups

20 butt kicks

Screams. Somewhere behind me. Abruptly silenced. The throaty growl of blasters. Damn it! These are Regulators. This is completely outside the law. I have no time to think and I need to work out what's happening. What my options are.

I make it to the cluster of buildings with my lungs burning. Vision blurry.

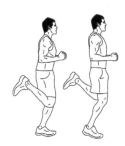

200 butt kicks

"Open up!" I yell and pound at the central one. Big armored steel door. I turn to look at one of the cameras positioned outside. "Take the kid!"

The door swings open on whisper-quiet hinges. Surreal quality adding to the nightmare. Inside it's darkness and rough hands seize me, pull me in. The door shuts again. Low bulbs instantly come to life. The contrast and sequence of events adds to the nightmare. Nothing feels real.

"Sef?" a voice I recognise.

I nod during my ascent. "The kid," I begin.

"He'll be OK,"

"What's happening?"

"Regulators. Corporation attack."

It doesn't make sense. Nothing makes sense. My eyes itch from the red dust. My head hurts. A lot. And now, as the adrenaline dials down, I think I can taste the red dust in my mouth.

"We're safe here," says someone.

He's wrong. We're not. I saw the Regulators outside. Saw the weapons they carried. I still hold a blaster in one hand. As if to punctuate my thoughts there is a massive blast blow to the door. It clangs with the noise of tortured metal, but holds.

People jostle me and I lose my footing. Fall to the floor on all fours.

"Sef!" the familiar voice again. I know the face but the name doesn't come to me. It occurs to me that no one knows me by that name here. The thought vanishes.

"Have you seen my wife?" a voice. More. They ask each other about family, friends, loved ones. The ones caught outside. The red dust.

Someone steps on my hand and I cry out. My voice is lost as another massive clang comes from the door.

I move instinctively, crawling on all fours, still. I get up as soon as I can and sprint for the back of the building, pushing through the press of bodies around me.

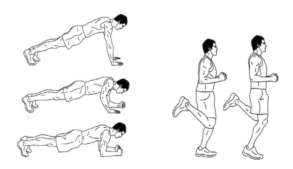

20 up and down planks and then 100 butt kicks

"Sef!" the voice calling me by a name it shouldn't. Not here. I don't look back. I feel like I want to die. I grit my teeth. Stand up. Begin to run.

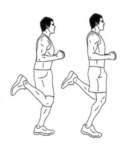

200 butt kicks

I reach the back of the structure just as there is one more massive clang. I am looking for a way out. My head hurts.

Luck more than anything else leads me to a service door. It's at the very back of the structure. Away from the crowd and the yells. It looks like an airlock except there is no need for airlocks on Orion. We're on a rock.

CLANG! The sound gets louder. CLANG!

My hands spin the wheel locks.

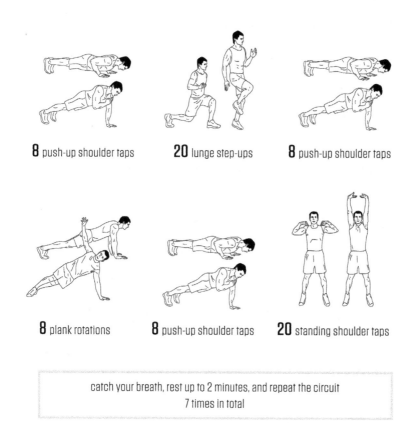

8 push-up shoulder taps   **20** lunge step-ups   **8** push-up shoulder taps

8 plank rotations   **8** push-up shoulder taps   **20** standing shoulder taps

catch your breath, rest up to 2 minutes, and repeat the circuit
7 times in total

I pull back the thick door step inside. Close it.

The floor beneath my feet vanishes.

CLANG! Above me. Bright light.

I fall. Darkness around me. It's hard to breathe and I realize
why there was an airlock. Some kind of pneumatic tube. A
means of transporting stuff around the colony buildings. I
brace myself for the impact.

It never comes. Hot, red air swirls around me. Red air? RED
AIR? My head hurts. I try to understand. I am still falling.
The structure I'd been in is no more. I feel more than see
the moment its molecules turn to dust. Banned weapons.
The Regulators using dematerialization bombs. Souped-up
versions of the blasters. My hand is still clutched around
mine.

Red dust everywhere. I can't breathe.

***

"SEF!" Reed's familiar voice breaks through to me. My eyes
blink and the red dust fades away.

"All those people," I groan. The pain in my head is worse.

"It's okay Sef, you're safe here," Reed's trying to be soothing. He's failing.

"They're all dead," I say. "Turned to dust,"

"It's OK," Reed says. He looks over his shoulder and someone I have never seen before appears on cue.

"I-" I try to get up. Fail. My head ... There's a dry touch to my neck. Something stings. Then. Nothing.

Chapter 20

Daylight. More pain. Less than before. OK.

"Where am I?" I blink to clear my eyes.

Ellie bends all solicitous over me. Ellie? What?

"You're safe," she says. "Been through some fever though."

I feel dehydrated. "How long-"

"Two weeks," she says. "You've been out for two weeks."

Hell! Two weeks. My brain is still reeling from my dream of the fate of Orion.

"What is this place?"

"It's a Sanctuary."

I groan.

Sanctuaries are neutral stations. They thrive on trade. They're armed to the teeth. Everything there costs something. It's not good for us to be here.

"Raynar?"

"He saved your life."

"I saved his,"

Ellie arches an eyebrow. "As sensitive and appreciative as ever, I see."

"Where are the others?"

"Negotiating."

"What?"

"Staying here is not without a cost."

Tell me something I don't know. I sit up. The pain... I need to stretch my muscles.

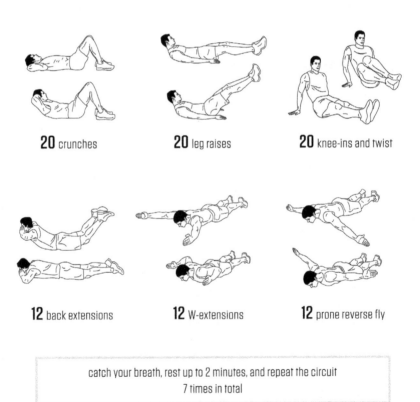

| 20 crunches | 20 leg raises | 20 knee-ins and twist |
| 12 back extensions | 12 W-extensions | 12 prone reverse fly |

catch your breath, rest up to 2 minutes, and repeat the circuit
7 times in total

Take in my surroundings. I am in a perfectly square white room. There is a bank of monitors on one side, all hooked up to my bed. The bed itself is white. White sheets. White pillows. I am dressed in some sort of white gown.

"My clothes?"

"I will get you some," Ellie walks away. Only then do I wonder A. why did we come to the Sanctuary and B. how come she's awake?

When Ellie returns with my clothes I notice they've been cleaned. "My blaster?"

"Gone. There is a strict no weapons policy here," she says.

"The Chimera?"

"Dead. Raynar turned it into dust," Ellie hides something in her voice that I can't identify.

We are, I guess, in a Healing Pod. Dedicated rooms staffed
by virtual medics. I'd heard of them but had never seen
the inside of one, until now. Outside, the surroundings are
decidedly less pristine. Ellie has to update something on
a screen before we can both leave the Pod. She talks as we
walk, filling me in.

"Raynar brought you to the bridge. You were bleeding badly,
your head looked hurt."

I remembered swirling Red Dust. Piles and piles of it getting
blown up into the air. Red Dust everywhere. My recurring
nightmare of Orion. I suppress the shiver that's beginning to
crawl down my spine.

"It still hurts," I say. I wonder how much of my nightmare is
real.

"You took some pretty serious damage. When Raynar
brought you, you were drifting in and out of consciousness.

We had to decide what to do."

"You could have left me."

"Reed wanted to. Tessa made him reconsider,"

I absorbed that piece of information. "And you?"

"Tessa managed to snap me out of my stasis. Then when we got here she had everything she needed to help me heal."

I nodded. There were still things that didn't make sense but at least I understood where we were and how we had got here.

"Take me to the others," I asked.

"You're just so predictable," Ellie smirked and herded me outside.

Sanctuaries are sophisticated stations. Everyone there has some kind of story. Some complex reason for their presence at a place where politics as usual do not compute.

To understand this consider that space is really big. Way bigger than anyone can imagine. Its vastness makes waystations, Sanctuaries necessary. But Sanctuaries are expensive to run and expensive to maintain. They provide little by way of profit if they were to be run that way. Corporations do not want to provide them.

Governments can't. A Sanctuary would constitute a governmental presence. It would have to be defended so a military outpost would be established. Governments don't have the clout to do that everywhere and they certainly don't have the money. The Corporations could, but there is no money in it for them. So it's left to private enterprise. Sanctuaries is the closest you'll get to entrepreneurs in space.

The private consortiums that set up and run them are backed, rumour has it, by space pirates and criminal clans, but no one has ever proven anything.

My head still aches a little and one side of my body feels like it's been through a metal press. Whatever they have been doing to me in the Healing Pod however seems to have helped. I can feel all my toes and fingers and my body moves just like before.

"This way," Ellie points to a backstreet.

Sanctuaries are like rabbit warrens. They start off small and grow big as need dictates. This makes them a sort of gigantic mental onion. New layers appear on top of the old ones, bolted on and joined by walkways, tunnels and pneumatic tubes. Ellie somehow seems to have mapped this out.

We go up ladder after ladder, cross one walkway after another until we get to a plateau of sorts.

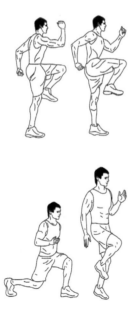

20 march steps

4 lunge step-ups

20 march steps

4 lunge step-ups

20 march steps

4 lunge step-ups

20 march steps

4 lunge step-ups

20 march steps

4 lunge step-ups

This place is crazy.

"We avoid drawing attention this way," Ellie says by way of explanation.

It's true. The few people we come across on the way are too busy with the pressure of their own lives to pay attention to us. We blend in. Just another two dwellers on a spinning chunk of metal, hanging in space.

"Why?" I ask her before we get to where the others are.

"Why what?"

"Why save me at all?"

She stops and looks at me, momentarily weighing her answer. Finally: "No choice."

"What?"

"There are Regulators after us. Don't know how. Or why. But we have to run and you might be the only one who can keep us alive long enough."

"Raynar is a Regulator." I say, puzzled.

"Well, there's a bounty out on his head too."

"What?" it's fast becoming my favorite word talking to
Ellie and I am beginning to dislike this shrinking of my
vocabulary.

"Reed intercepted a transmission. He was doing his usual
scans as we were trying to decide what to do next, looking for
the nearest place we could safely go to, when he came across
a high-end transmission. Full encryption. It's an all-out alert.
You, Raynar, Sam too apparently, though I guess she's now
gone. Me and Reed. We are a band of brothers and sisters
whether we want to or not, it seems."

It was hard to tell if she was serious. "OK,"

"OK,"

"So, we are negotiating for ...."

"Protection, extra ship armaments one or two fuel cells."

"I see."

I didn't but I couldn't tell her that. Something did not quite add up here but that was OK too. I would work it out.

***

The place where Raynar, Reed and Tessa are meeting the Sanctuary's negotiation team is all chrome and glass. The juxtaposition with the jerry-rigged layers we crossed to get there is not lost on me.

We're shown in by two goons in exoskeletons. Kinda puts you on edge when you have nothing but flesh and blood to work with, yourself.

"Ah, the recovering party," says one of the Sanctuary's negotiators as we enter. Is there an undertone of irony in his voice?

I sit next to Raynar, Ellie next to Tessa. "What have I missed?" I ask. There are six of them, sitting stone-faced across from us.

"The Sanctuary shakedown routine," growls Raynar and I begin to understand the undertone of irony I detected in the Sanctuary negotiator's voice.

"We prefer to call it bargaining," says the same negotiator that spoke before, but there's no rancor in his voice.

"They want our ship," explains Reed.

"Ah," I say. "We can't just yet swim through space," out of the corner of my eye I catch Ellie giggle before she remembers just how dire our situation is.

"We let you in and gave you medical assistance," the Sanctuary negotiator is talking again. He's the only one whose face is at all animated. The others might as well be automatons. They sit there looking at us.

As a psychological ploy it works. They add weight to everything said without shifting a muscle. But there is more here. I have seen this before and I know what it is. To test it I make a proposition.

"What if we leased you our ship instead? Let you use it for a specified length of time?" Raynar turns his head sharply to look at me and Reed and Tessa look crestfallen. I can't read quite what Ellie is thinking. My suggestion does the trick. I watch as the Sanctuary negotiator that has been talking smiles to hide the slow blink as he is thinking it over. Neural link. The team of six, in front of us, is talking to each other. They are studying us, analyzing our every move, and feeding suggestions to the talker in their midst.

"How would we work out what length of time is fair?" asks the talker eventually.

There are several options open to me now. When you know how someone works you understand the structure of their approach and you can disrupt it. I could have Reed try some of his magic and see if he can use his implants to intercept or disrupt the communication between the members of the Sanctuary's negotiating team, but that's risky. First of all it's an attack, however covert. Secondly, if it doesn't work we are in a pickle. Maybe not quite the same pickle as back there on the mining planet with the Cannibals, but a pickle nonetheless.

I choose to do something else entirely. "Regulators are after us," I say. I ignore the combined gasps of Ellie, Tessa, Reed and Raynar.

"You seem to have an unusual style of bargaining," the talker smiles strangely, "I can see now why they wanted you here."

"I'm not bargaining," I say, "Cards on the table. You want our ship. We can't give it to you. Yet we owe you for your help. Our heads are worth a lot, but you can't take them. Not without ceding Sanctuary status which then lays open all sorts of issues.

"What are you offering instead?"

"A trade. We each have skills. Use us for them. We will exchange know-how, help you upgrade your knowledge base." He is quiet and I know I am hitting home. Sanctuaries are like islands. Essentially isolated. Knowledge and skill sets is something they get only when people stay.

After a pause, "What kind of skills?"

"Weapons and tactics," I nod towards Raynar, "medical," I look at Tessa, "maybe we might even help you shorten that neural link communication gap," I point with my chin at Reed. I see the Sanctuary negotiator momentarily stiffen, then, a moment later relax. "You are interesting," he says at last. "I can see why they need you."

"Do we have a deal?" This time he doesn't even try to hide the fact that he is communicating with his colleagues.

"Yes, we do,' he says at last and reaching across the table offers me his open hand. "Name's Oscar," he says.

"Sef," I take it.

Chapter 21

After the trouble we had experienced, life on the Sanctuary was like a holiday. Raynar taught unarmed combat to the Sanctuary's troops. Weapons and tactics training, after that. Reed showed them how to shorten neural pulses without losing cohesion and clarity. Tessa had to hike over a mile each day to get to the lowest levels of the Sanctuary and talk to doctors there, help them upgrade their diagnostics.

Ellie was left alone to do Ellie things. And I ... I was left free to heal completely and wander across the Sanctuary talking to people and coming to grips with my nightmares.

Ugly memories of red dust still haunted me. As I got stronger and the pain from my head faded I found myself pondering the importance behind my red dust dreams. The shrieking of blasters and the undulating red mist left in the air.

"I like it here," Reed said after a few days. "These guys are really cool once you get them on your side."

We were at one of the restaurants. Restaurants! This place was amazing. Reed was busy working his way through a pile of grilled corn and mashed potatoes. We were drinking some local brew. Even Raynar was smiling.

"I am really sorry about Sam," I said to him, my voice purposefully low.

He nodded. "Yeah, she deserved better. She lost her brother at the Orion Massacre, you know."

"She did?"

"Yeah that's why she was always interested in it. Read those graphic novels all the time. Three Regulator ships blasted out of the sky. Over six squads disappeared. Turned into so much red, alongside all the miners. It was a disaster."

"What happened exactly?"

He shrugged. "No one knows for sure. The way we have it is the miners came under some kind of attack, called in for Regulator help per protocol. It took our ships over two days to get there, flying fast from a nearby orbital. We got there and we were attacked. Our forces wiped out. All ships destroyed. One ship stolen. We found just suits on the planet below. Blaster-scarred and scribbled with those words."

"Words?"

"Yeah. Red Reaper."

"I heard about that," Reed chips in, mouth half-full and chewing. He really has zero manners. "There was clandestine footage circulated all over the dark net. Grainy video of Regulator suits arrayed like trophies. Each one with 'Red Reaper' burnt on it. No bodies though. Just a planet full of red dust. Gross!"

Tessa is saying nothing. She's eating methodically, carefully chewing her food. Ellie is frowning. "Let's get back to work," I say and stand up to leave the table.

***

I see the device fly towards the already damaged structures below. Banned weapon. It is cigar shaped and metallic in nature. It hovers over the cluster of buildings below. It centers itself above them fins opening up to arrest its plummet and then, as its terrible payload begins to react, it turns into a miniature strobe of death.

White flashes emanate from it. Wherever they touch steel and concrete, wood and glass heat up, melt, disintegrate. But the worst thing occurs on flesh and blood. The hundreds of miners that had sought refuge below. As the roof of their building evaporates, the white flashes continue. Touch their bodies, heads. They rise up like ghosts in the mist. Silent. Like a well coordinated dance troupe they all simmer and then vanish. Swirling red piles left behind.

"Sef!" the familiar voice cuts through to me. The tableau disintegrates and I become aware of the sweat drenching me.

"Wake up!". It's Ellie.

***

"You have to go," this from Oscar. We are in a suite like the one we used to negotiate in, but much smaller. No goons this time.

"Regulators are here," says Raynar. He's there ahead of us. There is some commotion and Tessa comes running in too. Reed two steps behind her.

"Great!" I am already out of breath. "You're a neutral station. Sanctuary is to be respected." I say to Oscar. He looks a little dubious. He's alone in this room, the five colleagues he showed up with during our negotiating are not here and, without them I am not sure he can see everything the way I can. It's not that he's not smart but when you're used to -

"We've spoken to their commander," he says. The momentary blink before he speaks. Of course. They don't need proximity for the neural connection to work. I wonder just what the range of it is. "A Captain Jackal,"

Raynar lets out a groan.

"You know him?" I enquire.

"Piece of work. He's barely Regulator. They only assign him the worst cases."

I am not wholly convinced of Regulator piousness. I remember Orion. "So?"

"He's not here to talk," Raynar says.

"This is Sanctuary," I repeat like an idiot.

"Exactly," Oscar says. He's looking at me pointedly, waiting patiently for me to make the connection. Sanctuary. You don't violate Sanctuary and expect to get away with it. It creates all sorts of problems. Major problems. No Corp or Regulator ship would ever be able to find assistance in a Sanctuary, unless - they can see the thought unfold in my face.

"Orion all over again," I say.

"What do you know about Orion?" Tessa asks, then catches herself.

"Orion was the Red Reaper's work," says Raynar abstractly. His mind is focused elsewhere.

"Let the comms through," I say to Oscar. We are all a little frazzled. Sanctuary life had began to grow on us a little. Oscar nods to a technician and the table in front of us projects a hologram.

Captain Jackal, surprisingly, does not look like a four-legged, pointy-nosed, fur-covered animal from Terra's past. So there must be another reason they call him that. "Captain," I say. Cameras in the room feed our images back to him. The on-lens AI stitches together the visuals allowing him to feel like he is really there, standing in the middle of our table, with us all around.

"Oscar," he acknowledges Oscar. No titles or niceties. OK. That sets the tone. "Give us the girl." Just like that. Out of the corner of my eye I see Ellie shrink into herself a little.

"Captain Jackal, we've not met before," says Oscar.

"The girl," Captain Jackal repeats as if he hasn't heard a word.

"Ellie?" I ask.

His eyes turn to me. Scan me with some scorn. Dismiss me. Well, well.

"Yeah, hand her over." He says.

"Or?"

Oscar tries to cut me off. Too late.

"You do not want us to come in." OK. A threat. Maybe. Perhaps not the same scale as Orion. Maybe it is though.

"You have one hour," he cuts off. Just like that.

"I don't think he's kidding," Reed says in his understated way.

Oscar is pacing the room now, conferring with his counterparts. I briefly wonder what it's like to have such close connection with others. Then I realize that once again here I am, fighting to survive. It was all meant to be over by now. I should have been at the Hub and then Eden. It makes me angry and I choke it down. Practice deep breathing until the red mist clears from my eyes.

My mind is racing to formulate a plan. Regulator ships are well armed but then so are Sanctuaries.

"Hurry, we have very little time!" Oscar has finished discussing whatever discussion he was sharing with his neurally connected counterparts. And it appears they've reached a decision.

We are all off running.

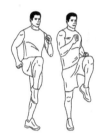

100 high knees

We climb down some shafts, following Oscar, slide down some tubes, then up some ladders.

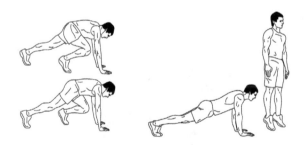

60 climbers and then **20** basic burpees (no push-ups)

More ladders.

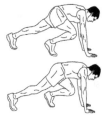

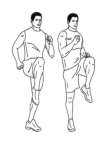

10 climbers

20 high knees

10 climbers

20 high knees

10 climbers

20 high knees

10 climbers

20 high knees

10 climbers

20 high knees

And more.

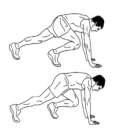

100 climbers

We are all sweating.

"These are not passages everyone knows," says Oscar.

We are moving and I am thinking. My brain works best when I am exercising and all the physical activity moves it into high gear.

"How much further?" I ask.

"Ten minutes," says Oscar.

The ten minutes go fast.

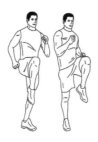

200 high knees

The climbs and slides and climbs again take us to the service tunnel leading to the docks.

"Your ship is ready to go," says Oscar, "we've been testing all systems and have enhanced your weaponry."

"Our stuff?" says Tessa. There is real panic in her voice.

"We've had most of it brought onboard."

"Thank you!" I see the relief on her face.

I am sure the Regulators are monitoring the Sanctuary so we can't go through the usual hot launch sequence. We uncouple from the station and let the drift take us away, its bulk hiding us from the Regulator ship on the other side.

"I have everything on power down," Reed says.

He's not kidding. Even the temperature is low. We all have to do jumping exercises to keep warm.

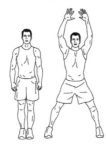

50 jumping jacks

Thanks to the alacrity at which Oscar responded we have a full thirty minutes before the deadline Captain Jackal issued is over.

"Will they be OK?" Ellie voices everyone's anxiety. We've all come to like and respect the Sanctuary folks.

"With us away there is nothing that the Regulators can do," says Raynar.

We busy ourselves with work to help keep us warm. Raynar is stacking provisions, lifting the heavy metal boxes like they weigh nothing. Reed is jogging on the spot while working at his station. Ellie and Tessa are reorganizing the ship's sick bay and I, I need to think.

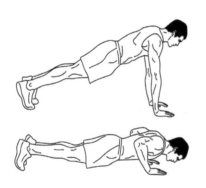

10 push-ups

catch your breath

10 push-ups

catch your breath

10 push-ups

catch your breath

10 push-ups

catch your breath

10 push-ups

Mentally I am keeping track of everything. As my body works and its temperature rises I can see the patterns that form. How dots, connected, begin to present a very specific picture. I am not sure I fully understand it, but what I see in my mind's eye fits. I think I know how the Regulators found us at the Sanctuary.

I am in the process of considering how to best test my theory when a deep shudder runs through the ship and knocks me off my feet. Reed barely has time to grab onto something and Raynar is almost crashed by one of the heavy boxes he's moved as it falls off before he can secure it.

"What was that?" I ask.

Reed is going through his panel. Hands flicking from switch to switch while part of him, the part that's full of implants, whispers quietly to the ship's instrumentation.

"No!" he gasps.

"What?"

"The Sanctuary. It - ..... It's not there anymore!"

Tessa and Ellie have come running from their tasks in sick bay to hear him as he says that. Ellie lets out a low gasp.

"Are you sure?"

"I've checked twice. It's gone."

I consider the banned weapons used to take out a space station. There was no need for the Regulators to do that. I can see why Captain Jackal has the reputation he has.

"Have they spotted us?" I ask. Without the station's bulk hiding us the Regulator ship could easily spot us, I think.

"No. They can't." says Reed. "We're still running cold. The space between us and them is now full of debris."

We continue to drift, slowly through space. A ship running cold. And my anger boiling hot.

Chapter 22

Ellie was in tears. The rest of us were silent. Cut up.

The moment we made a safe distance, Reed fired up our ship's engines and we became lost in space. One more non-descript dot in a sea of darkness punctuated by non-descript dots.

"I am running the ship on essential power only," Reed announced. "That way we save fuel plus our signature is mostly hidden."

That was fine. I run around the outside of the deck to keep warm. I do push ups in my room, to help me think. The rest do their own thing too. The ship, in sadness, becomes a hive of activity, each of us honing our body because we have little else to do and no other way to channel our feelings.

"I need to get to my dad," Ellie's eyes were red with tears. Her breathing interspersed with sobs. "I need to get to Andromeda 6."

Just like that we are full circle again. I am back on the loading dock of GT-701 contemplating an easy passage to a new life and Ellie is a passenger on a nondescript cargo ship that's going to become the focal point of a Regulator boarding party.

"It's not safe,"

"I still need to get there."

Great. I remind her of the Regulators who came on board the cargo ship. They most likely knew where she was going. To even try to get to Andromeda 6 is to walk into a Regulator trap. They don't really need to find us and hunt us down. All they have to do is wait and scoop us up when we appear.

Ellie is persistent. "If I reach out to my uncle, he'll know what to do," she says. I veto it. The Regulators are likely to be monitoring every channel. Raynar agrees. So does Tessa. Only Reed remains silent. Ellie tries begging me. I am not going to budge.

"Perhaps there is a way," Reed volunteers at last.

"I'm listening,"

"There is a group of erm, shall we say entities, we can reach out to." He describes the Wired to us. A fringe group, leaving out in space. More machine than human. They could get a secure message to anyone, anywhere.

I have never heard of them, but then again they don't sound like the kind of beings likely to cross my path. "How do we contact them?" I ask.

"That's easy. I shall sent out a subspace message on a particular frequency. Something that normal instrumentation is likely to see only as background space radiation. The Wired will pick it up. Get back to us."

It seems the easiest thing in the world. "What's the catch?"

Reed hesitates. Then: "They're a bit … erm, quirky shall we say?"

Quirky? That coming from Reed sounds quirky in itself.

"There's no telling what's important to them. They will only tell us once."

"And it's secure?" this from Raynar.

"Totally."

"Ok," I say. "Do it. Send them a message."

I watch Reed's eyes glaze over as his mind goes elsewhere. I can't help wondering just what it must be like to live inside his body, part of it augmented with all sorts of internal circuitry. The sensorium he experiences must be so different to the rest of us I actually wonder if he is entirely human.

"Done," he announces. His eyes blink rapidly, clearing. He refocuses. "I have a location. We are to meet them there."

'There' - turns out to be an old disused communications relay station. These used to be vital at one stage when mining planets were closer together and comms tech was more primitive. Turns out they were vulnerable to space radiation, burning out just when you needed them most. They were abandoned and fell into disuse when subspace communication was made possible via Hilbert space configuration.

"Some of them are still around," Reed explains. It's like he just read my thoughts. "They're still used to communicate through, erm ... not quite the way you think."

He doesn't explain anything else and now I am thinking that all of this is way too easy.

We fly through space without incident. I take some time to talk to Ellie.

"I will get a message to your uncle," I say, "see also if he has an update on your dad's whereabouts. But if I sense anything's wrong you will do exactly what I say."

She's not impressed, but what choice does she have? I watch Reed flick through his dials and I realize that at a certain level he must be the closest thing to Oscar with his neurally linked pals, there is. Who is he in communication with, I wonder.

My eyes flit over the other two occupants of the deck. Raynar is practicing drawing the blaster. He puts it in the holster by his side and then with a flick of his wrist it appears in his hand. He's fast.

Tessa is busy writing down notes on an old style tablet. She's using a stylus for that and one of the alphanumeric alphabets. The moment she completes each paragraph the tablet converts it into binary and stores it in an internal archive. I find it fascinating that she's working at a time like this.

I bring my mind back to what we are doing and I wonder at just where I ended up. I am as far from my original destination and intent as any human can possibly get.

"I am a little derailed," I say to no one in particular. There is no point in feeling sorry about yourself. Everything is a choice and in getting to this point, here, I certainly made plenty of them. I could have left Ellie to the Regulators, a long time ago.

I have learnt to live with my choices. I quietly take myself off to one side, away from the others. I go through a punishing round of upper body strength exercises and stretching. The pain of the physical effort involved grounds me. It makes me forget how sorry I feel and I focus, again, on the life force I sense inside me. The thing that makes me who I am.

By the time I finish, drenched in sweat, we are almost there. I get to Raynar. "Hey," I say.

"Hey," he returns. He was watching me exercise.

"About Orion,"

"Yeah?"

"I was wondering. If no one survived, how do the Regulators know what really happened?"

He thinks about that one for a sec. Shrugs. "Dunno. Cameras maybe?"

"Well, they must have had something to create the narrative." I persist.

"Yeah I guess. Didn't really think about it before."

"We're here." Reed announces.

Our destination is like a tin can hanging in space. It's rectangular. As large as a house. Immobile, which means no gravity.

Reed explains how it works to us and it sounds crazy already.

"There's no getting any closer than now," he says, "These things have all sorts of field force protections because they were so easy to sabotage. We shall have to spacewalk, get to it. Get inside. "There is telemetry gear we can plug into, right there. You can talk directly to the Wired through your suit mic," he explains.

I would much rather do it from inside the ship but there is no way this can happen. As you might have guessed, I am no big fan of spacewalks. They leave you too vulnerable, especially when you don't really know what you're walking into. Still, I reason to myself, whoever the Wired may be, whatever they may be, they need something from us, that's not our lives, otherwise it would be much easier to sabotage our ship or simply broadcast our presence to Regulators. The thought calms me down a little.

"I will be with you every step of the way, from here." Reed says, he points to the instrument console.

It's no consolation. Once again I find myself stepping from an airlock into the cold darkness of space. I use my suit jet to aim for the comms relay station. It's actually bigger than it looked from the ship. I revise my opinion upwards. About as big as ten houses.

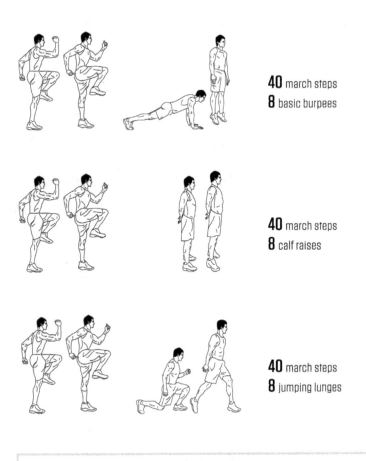

40 march steps
8 basic burpees

40 march steps
8 calf raises

40 march steps
8 jumping lunges

catch your breath, rest up to 2 minutes, and repeat the circuit
7 times in total

"Sef, you're approaching too fast. Ease on the jets." Reed's voice in my ear sounds reassuring. I follow his instructions adjusting for balance as well as speed.

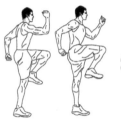

200 march steps

Once on the relay station I get into a small housing. There are banks of crude equipment I don't recognize all along one wall. Reed guides me expertly to one of them. Tells me what to do. It's not complicated but without his guidance I would never have done it.

"OK, Sef, you're in." He says.

For the briefest moment there is nothing. Then a small jolt like a current and my helmet's visor turns into a display. I see shadowy figures, five, six, maybe more. They are bunched together, leaning forward. Straining to see me.

"Is this VR?" I ask.

"Kinda," says one. The tone is sibilant. I sense it more than hear it. I realize it's bone induction. The sound is coming through the instrumentation.

I am not sure how to begin. "I - well, thank you for accepting our request. I was going to - "

"We shall let the uncle know the girl is alive. Wants to meet." They cut me off.

Did Reed tell them already, I wonder.

"No." They say. "We read your thoughts."

Damn! Immediately I regret the reaction. I try to blank my mind, but realize I am not quite sure how.

"Interesting," says one of them.

"What?"

"We have a condition for our help."

Of course. I stop any other thought from articulating. Damn telepaths! Oh -

They chuckle. "You're funny."

"Glad I amuse you."

They tell me the request. What they want of me. Reed said they were weird. He wasn't kidding. The display in front of my eyes vanishes just as suddenly as it had appeared.

"Well?" Reed's voice cuts in anxiously. "Are you OK?"

"Why wouldn't I be?"

"We lost you there for a moment. We were getting worried."
"Ah, they blocked you," I say. "They will get the message to the uncle."

"You're starting back then?"

"Not yet. There is something I have to do first." I wait, I know they are listening. Reed's waiting also. "I need to run a maze."

Silence. Then: "Come again."

"A maze. They want me to run a maze."

"Where?"

"Here. In space." More silence. To be expected really. I take pity on Reed. "There is a maze inside the structure apparently. They want me to run it."

"Like a rat?" Reed says.

It makes me wonder if he does have a sense of humor after all.

"They've given me a code. It opens the airlock. I run the maze. Come out. Get suited up. Get back. Easy." I say.

"You'll have no comms to keep in contact with us." He's right. Then again the Wired did cut me off while they were talking to me. I point this out.

"OK, Sef. Be careful."

Yeah, right. Like a maze run in space is something you can ever really prepare for.

I punch in the code and get to the airlock. Take off the bulky suit. I strip to my underwear. Step through. Perversely enough it's warm inside the structure. It's dimly lit but my eyes adjust quickly. I look at the maze beginning before me. There is a red digital counter to my right. I know the moment I enter the maze it will begin counting down.

"Beat the countdown." The Wired said. No mention of how long or short it might be. I assumed they are reasonable. My death holds no meaning to them. Still, there will be little time to dally.

"Ok Sef." I tell myself. "Time to prove you're as good as you think you are." I take one last deep, measured breath and then I am off and running. Arms pumping and knees rising as I power through the maze, eyes and brain working frantically, solving the puzzle on the go.

The oxygen inside the structure tastes stale. As I gulp it down
my lungs are burning and I wonder briefly if it is enough.
Time seems to slow down. The walls of the maze stretch
endlessly. I take turn after turn. Mark walls down with my
mind, remembering angles and the way the shadows bounce
off them.

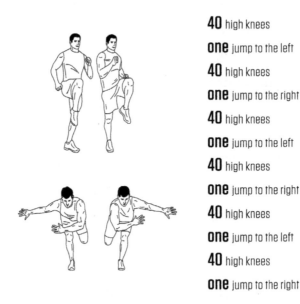

40 high knees
one jump to the left
40 high knees
one jump to the right
40 high knees
one jump to the left
40 high knees
one jump to the right
40 high knees
one jump to the left
40 high knees
one jump to the right

Then, just when I think I can go on no more. Just when
it feels like the oxygen has run out. I get to the end. I am
drenched in sweat.

It takes me some time to get dressed again. Work my way through the airlock. Get back to the ship. When I get there I am exhausted.

"We got word from them." Reed says while Raynar is helping me take my suit off. "The message went through. Leonidas Ri. Ellie's uncle will be waiting at the Hub. Dock 17."

Finally.

Chapter 23

The Hub is my destination. It has always been my destination. From there I will disappear. Ellie's uncle couldn't have chosen a better location.

"We can't get there directly," I say, but that's not what I mean. Of course we can just fly in and touch down. I can't however. There are things I need to take care of. Before I disappear, loose ends. "You'll put me down in the dunes, way outside the inhabited area."

The Hub is surrounded by dunes. Desert really. It's what makes it so attractive. Beyond the fact that it's easy to defend because land assaults are near impossible, it also allows it to concentrate the population within its borders. Think of the Hub as your biggest planetary Metropolis and you're not even close.

Nearly 30 million people live in one giant city on a planet that has the same name. Almost the same name. Cartographers added "1" so the Hub, to be pedantic, is within Hub-1. And Hub-1 is a desert planet whose main industry is the massive trade carried out within its megacity.

Because of where it is ships take off for the outer planets, be they mines or colonies. Its light gravity and thin atmosphere, all the things that so tax off-worlders, make it perfect for ships to land and take off in the most economic fashion possible.

The dunes have some other attractions, too. For me at least.

Reed looks at me like I have gone crazy. "You're not coming with us?"

"Nope. Ellie will get into her uncle's hands. Raynar here will be looking for some freelance outfit to join, I guess, and you will do whatever it is you do. I have to get outta here."

Finally, I am thinking. I am getting things back on track.

"Can I come with you?" Tessa asks.

I look at her speculatively for a moment. Then: "Sure."

"There's a scientific weather station at the very heart of the desert." She says. "I've never had time to pay them a visit. This is the perfect opportunity."

I nod. I can see Ellie look a little crestfallen. It occurs to me that the kid had thought we were all one big team for life. No such luck. Besides, the loose ends. I need to tie them. Urgently.

"Can you kill all ship comms for now?" I ask Reed.

"Everything?"

"Everything."

He doesn't ask why. He does something to the switches on his console and his eyes also glaze briefly as he activates some code and then looks at me: "Done".

I nod my thanks.

"Precautions?" Raynar asks. The others wait to hear what I will say.

"Comms are difficult to hide. If we get scanned, comms is the only signature we can't disguise."

"That's true," Reed agrees.

"So comms blackout until you guys get to the Hub."

Reed takes it in his stride. I am really going to miss him. "Ok," he says.

Dune landings are a little rough. We have about an hour before we get where we need to and I use the time to limber up. The activity engages my body and frees my mind. I take the time to run through everything from the beginning. The ship, the Regulators, the girl, the Cannibals, Tessa, the Ghost Ship, the Chimeras. What should have been a routine flight to a paradise planet has ended up being a nightmare.

The thinking time does me good. I know exactly what I need to do next.

"Strap in," Reed says over the intercom and we all take landing positions.

He brings the ship down gently. The sand gives a little when we land but that's about it.

"The coordinates you asked for," he says. I thank him.

I shake Raynar's hand. "Take care of yourself," he says gruffly.

"It was a hell of a ride," I say back.

Lastly I hug Ellie. I don't know why. I have come to really like her. "Be careful," I say.

"You too."

That's it. Goodbyes are terrible. I grab my backpack. Look at Tessa. She has a couple of massive backpacks she is struggling with. "Is the scientific station far?" I ask. I already know the answer to that one.

"Two clicks East," she says.

"I will help you get there," I volunteer, waving away her protest.

We both watch the ship take off. I shoulder one of her backpacks. It weighs a ton. She takes the other. It's amazing she managed to get so much stuff in the short time we rescued her from the Cannibals.

"What will you do next?" I ask as we walk.

"It depends. I am a geneticist. There's always need for my skills with the Corporations."

It's the first time she said what kind of medical doctor she was and I absorb it. Nod to myself.

"And you? Where will you go?"

"Eden," I say.

"Eden?" She looks surprised. "That's an expensive planet to be on."

"I have money."

"That much?"

"Yep."

Walking on sand is exhausting. Especially if you're carrying weight which we both did. Tessa's backpack that I was carrying was heavy enough for the straps to feel like they were biting into my shoulder.

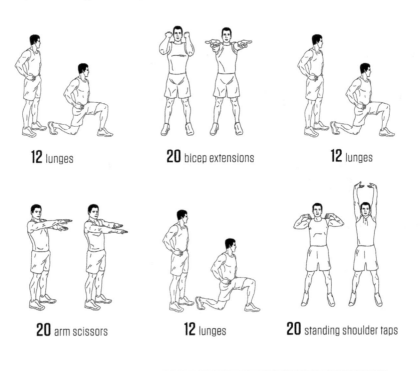

12 lunges   **20** bicep extensions   **12** lunges

20 arm scissors   **12** lunges   **20** standing shoulder taps

catch your breath, rest up to 2 minutes, and repeat the circuit
7 times in total

"Do you want to stop for a quick break? There is some shade over there," Tessa points to some jutting rocks. They provide some respite from the sun and the reflected heat.

"Sure."

We stop and put down our backpacks. With my left hand I rub my right shoulder where Tessa's backpack that I am carrying has bitten into it. It itches.

"Water?" Tessa offers me her water bottle. I decline. Take a sip from mine.

She looks at me with amusement on her face. Deliberately she unscrews her water bottle. Eyes on me she leans back and takes a long sip. Her eyes play over my frame. She can see my right hand is near the blaster at my waist.

"How long have you known?" she finally asks.

There. Just like that. "A few days. Since the attack at the Sanctuary," I say, "It didn't make sense. How the Regulators found us. And then everything else did."

"Just that?" she asks.

"Well, no. There were other things. Small. It all added up.
The fact that you were down on the Cannibal planet. Your
team died but you didn't. You were there to get specimens
and things went wrong. On the Ghost Ship you knew exactly
where to go for medical supplies. The place I found you
in wasn't even on the schematics. Yet you knew your way
around it."

"I thought I stumbled there, but we were running out of
time. The Chimeras were running around."

"Yeah, you knew." I say. "And you made Reed save me.
That made no sense. Plus you had access to comms at the
Sanctuary. Those Regulators didn't just stumble across us."

"Well, well, well." She appears unfazed and I draw my blaster
out of instinct. Her eyes do not even track it. "Not bad for the
legendary Red Reaper."

If I am surprised, I hide it.

"Orion had no survivors," she says. "I know that because we got there within a whisker of the departure of one of our ships. The only one of our ships sent there that made it out intact. Minus its crew of course. We found those planetside. All dead. How you managed to clock up such an impressive body count against Regulators is beyond me, but clearly you have the knack."

"What do you want with me?" I ask.

"Direct. Your Red Reaper reputation does not do you justice. I have looked at your genetics of course. Chimeras require the right raw material. A higher baseline than usual. You are exactly what I am looking for. You will be magnificent."

She makes no attempt to hide her plan. I bring the blaster up in line with her face.

"Ah, you thought I wouldn't plan this?"

I look at her. Try hard to think. Her name escapes me. I look at the blaster in my hand, suddenly heavy. It begins to fall. I try to raise it in vain. "How?" I manage.

"The backpack," she says with a smile. "The strap,"

I remember the roughness of the strap. Whatever soporific was there, to be absorbed by my skin.

She leans forward and takes the blaster out of my suddenly nerveless fingers. "Just in case you get any ideas," she smiles. "The guys at the station will take good care of you."

I cannot move, but out of the corner of my eye I can see approaching shapes.

"I will take care of your friends. Don't really care about them but the reward for the girl could come in handy. Besides, her genetics are surprising. She'll make an amusing baby Chimera."

I open my mouth but no sound comes out.

"Save your strength Red Reaper," she says mockingly, "you're gonna need it where you're going."

Chapter 24

"I don't understand the biometric readings on this one. He comes out clean every time I scan him," says one of the techs to the others.

I am dead meat. Tessa's soporific worked. I am left paralyzed. Muscles locked. Only the blink response working. And my brain, of course. I am thinking furiously. If thoughts had weight these three goons that carried me the rest of the way to their little science station would now be flat as pancakes.

I long for anger. Hate. The red mist that envelops me when
I am triggered. I dredge up everything I can. Orion, white
flashes and swirling flakes of red dust. Captain Jackal and
the casual way he destroyed the Sanctuary. He had to leave
no witnesses behind. Regulators running errands, hunting
a kid. Xelium. Mining colonies. Everything revolves around
energy. Fuel. Space itself could go cold and dark without
that. Just like I was inside. I wonder what it is she's given
me. What side-effects it will have. Not that it matters. They
have me.

It makes me laugh. The Red Reaper caught just like that.
Thought I'd covered every possible angle. Had worked the
puzzle out in my head. While Xelium was getting scarcer
and an energy crisis was coming, Corps were muscling
in, securing strongholds and supply. And beefing up their
weapon stockpiles. Banned energy weapons and experiments
in exotic, lethal life forms.

What a world we have managed to create. I think. The
universe has a sense of irony. I am on the Hub. I am where
I wanted to get to. From here I can catch a ship to Eden.
Disappear forever.

"Tessa said he's muscle for hire. Bio-engineered background to hide. Some top-notch hitman. Goes by the name of Red Reaper."

Their mention of Tessa's name snaps my attention back to the present.

"Red Reaper? The butcher of Orion?"

"Yep, the same."

I blink. My way of grinning right now. 'Butcher of Orion' - hah, in a way they're right. Partially right. I butchered the Regulator goons that had been sent to Orion. The real butchering had been done by them. But it's my word against theirs, or rather. My word, only. I am the only one who walked away from that one alive and I did not take pictures, shoot videos or create handy little narratives to tell the other mining planets.

"Ok, hotshot," I tell myself. The voice inside my head sounds clear and strong. It's only my body I can't move it seems. "How do we get out of this?"

Tessa blindsided me all along. I didn't see her for who she was down at the Cannibal planet and the signs were all there. The same little telltale signs that kept piling up. Adding up to a picture I saw only the last moment. You only see what you look at.

The thought gives me an idea. I first listen to the goons. They've got me on a gurney, inside their science station which clearly does not collect weather data. I am paralyzed so they haven't bothered strapping me down. Big mistake on their part, but only if I stop being paralyzed.

"We're to run a complete genome sequence on this one. Tessa thinks that we may have found our perfect host for gene splicing."

"A Chimera we can control? Yeah, that's what she said."

"Do we need the body kept alive or just the genes?"

"She didn't say. At the moment there is no danger. The paralyzing agent she used is not going to wear off any time soon."

Right. Ok. Except. Paralyzing agents work in one of two ways: They disrupt the brain, stop the neurons that control locomotion from functioning. You can will your body to do something but without the brain making it happen, it just won't. That's one of the reasons drunks have trouble standing up sometimes. Ethanol is the intoxicating part of alcohol and its molecules are so small that they can actually pass into the gaps between brain cells. There it can interfere with the neurotransmitters that enable all the brain's activities.

Or, they disrupt the muscles. Stop the nerve receptors from receiving the biochemical messengers that make them contract. A muscle contraction consists of a series of repeated events. First, calcium triggers a change in the shape of troponin and reveals the myosin-binding sites of actin beneath tropomyosin. Then, the myosin heads bind to actin and cause the actin filaments to slide. The cycle is repeated. The muscle contracts.

Relaxation occurs when stimulation of the nerve stops. Calcium is then pumped back into the sarcoplasmic reticulum breaking the link between actin and myosin. Actin and myosin return to their unbound state causing the muscle to relax.

I could think really clearly so what Tessa had given me was a muscle relaxant as opposed to a neural inhibitor. That was her mistake. The muscle relaxant she'd put in my bloodstream was blocking actin and myosin. Anything in the bloodstream is subject to metabolizing. Right now I was inert, but if I got my muscles to fire up it would speed up the process via which my bloodstream would get flushed and my muscles would be active again.

I didn't become the Red Reaper, the most feared assassin in the Galaxy by taking origami classes, though, I have very fond memories of origami. It helps me relax after a job. I know that visualization enhances neural pathways in the brain so it's easier for the nervous system to activate those muscles in real life. This gives me my plan. From the brain's perspective an intense, imaginary workout is no different to a real one.

While the lab rats are discussing protocols and the best way to sequence my DNA, I take deep even breaths, oxygenating my brain and body and further increasing my metabolic rate. In my mind, I visualize in very precise, clear detail, the hardest possible workout I can do. Already light beads of sweat begin to form at my temples.

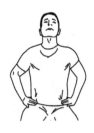

take 10 deep breaths

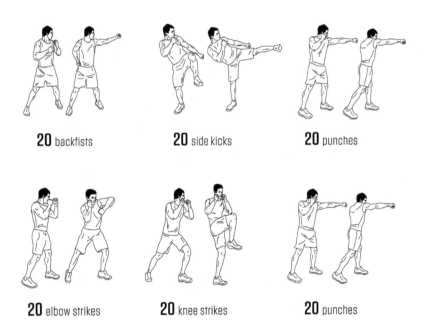

20 backfists

20 side kicks

20 punches

20 elbow strikes

20 knee strikes

20 punches

catch your breath, rest up to 2 minutes, and repeat the circuit
7 times in total

***

Plumes of smoke rise like heralds from the sand dunes behind me. I walk with purposeful strides going over the dune in front of me and down the other side, backpack over one shoulder.

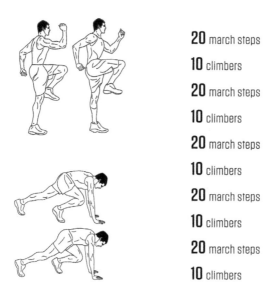

20 march steps

10 climbers

20 march steps

10 climbers

20 march steps

10 climbers

20 march steps

10 climbers

20 march steps

10 climbers

I am already tired. Exhausted actually and this, additional physical activity makes me sweat even more. But it flushes whatever remnants of paralyzing agent were left in my bloodstream. I feel the most clear-headed I have felt for a long time. My mind feels free, as if a weight has lifted off it and my body works like the finely-tuned biomachine that it is.

Can't say the same for the lab rats I left behind. They were so surprised to see me get up from the gurney they barely put up a fight. I trashed the lab and set the entire station on fire for good measure. Messed up some valuable scientific data in the process, I am sure.

So now, I am heading for the dune transporter over the dune I am climbing.

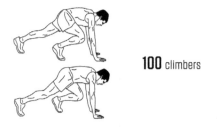

100 climbers

Heavy machine with wide caterpillar tracks that travel over the desert sand with incredible ease. I have a rendezvous with Tessa and a one-way ticket out of the Hub and I can't wait for either.

Chapter 25

The Hub is not the place to be. It is the only place to be on Hub-1, which means that finding anyone on it is a case of resources.

I've been to the Hub many times. And I know exactly where to go. I stop at a local store first and purchase a desert hoodie. They are, as the name suggests, based on a hoody of old except they are full body length coats with a hood, made out of a synth material that stops static, water and sand, in that order.

I also buy a new pair of desert boots. Heavy leather, buckles all the way to mid thigh. They armour your feet. The steel mesh surrounding them, just beneath the leather provides protection without adding too much weight. Where I am going now I am going to need them. A heavy pair of desert gloves, of similar design to the boots complete my purchase.

Kitted out I am now as invisible as it is possible for one person to be in the Hub. Eagle-eye cameras watch everything. Algorithms scan faces, clothes, height, gait. Catalogue everything. Flag up potential problems before they surface. Hub Regulators take care of the rest.

I am not keen to meet them now. I have work to do and time is against me.

I have no idea just how much of a headstart Tessa really has. She may not necessarily have been in a hurry. After all, she had got what she wanted and captured the Red Reaper in the process. Given the way she had been able to commandeer the lab rats at the now defunct scientific station my guess is she is no ordinary researcher. She has to be the leader of some corporate bio-weapons procurement program, which means she has means and clout.

The question is how much does she want to advertise her presence here, now? And mine.

My outfit is non-descript. Replicated by hundreds, maybe thousands of dwellers across the Hub. In plain sight, dressed like this, I can pass unnoticed. Just another stiff on some business in one of the Galaxy's most heavily populated commercial centers.

Alrighty then. I choose to walk than take any transport. The crowds hide me better and by not having to provide ID of any kind I am off the grid. Tessa may have been thorough. My new biochip info may be, by now, on some Corporate database, awaiting processing. I want to trigger as few alarms as possible.

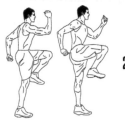

200 march steps

I melt through the crowds. Boots muting the contact with the ground, making my every step feel like I am invincible. Eventually I get to a place I know. I've been careful all this time. Doubling back and forth in what turned a mile-long journey into a distance that is several times that. No one's really paying attention to me, or tailing me.

Snug's shop is in an alley, just across from where I am standing. I careful check to make sure no one is really watching and then, casually, cross the street and melt in the alley at the side of it. Snug's shop has a bio-reader. I palm it. It hums. The door slides open. I am in.

That easy.

Now for the hard stuff.

"Snug", I throw back my hood.

Snug is a leech. He leeches off the need of others. Sure he provides a service but he does so on a sliding scale. The greater your need, the more expensive the service gets. You get the picture.

"You!" he recognizes me instantly. His surprise telling me everything I need to know. I catch the nod he gives to the muscle goons sitting on either side of the door behind me and I roll into action.

I sidekick the first.

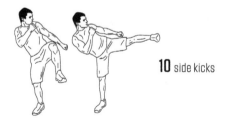

10 side kicks

Feel the satisfying crunch of solid contact of steel on ribs as my boot hits his side. He cries out and falls back, momentarily stunned and I catch the second one, as he moves forward, with elbow strikes. Quick swipes, one, two, three. He throws up his arms, defending but it's already too late for him. The steel-meshed gloves come into play.

Lights out.

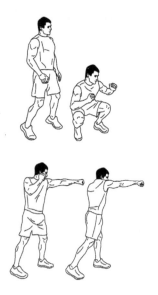

2 squats
20 punches
2 squats
20 punches
2 squats
20 punches
2 squats
20 punches
2 squats
20 punches

His friend has recovered from the kick. I kick again. This time to the head.

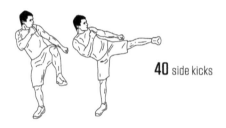

40 side kicks

He instinctively drops his arms, protecting his injured ribs. It leaves him wide open. His eyes roll back and he's unconscious before his head hits the floor.

I am through playing nice.

"No, wait!" Snug begins but already I am reaching. I don't put full force behind each punch. I want him to be awake. But clearly steel mesh gloves and human face flesh are not a good combination when any kind of force is involved.

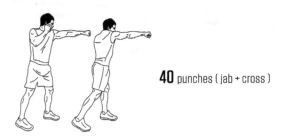

40 punches (jab + cross)

After the third blow he goes limp. "Please," he whimpers and I stop.

"Tell me why you thought I was dead," I say and he stiffens with alarm. "Don't lie."

"Ok, Ok. Stop hitting me! That scientist woman. The one with the attitude, she's been here to get the latest intel. She told me all about you. I didn't believe her. Really I didn't, especially when she said you're called Sef. Like you would ever use that name. But then she had blood samples she needed coded fast and transmitted. Skin cells. I thought she was for real. I really did. I had no choice. She had Regulators with her."

Snug stops talking and looks at me. There is blood leaking out his nose, the left eyebrow. His lip. And truth coming out his mouth.

"Ok," I let him go. "What did she want?"

"To find a group. Two men and a girl."

"Where are they?"

"Hanging around Hangar 9 as of three hours ago. Dock 17. Waiting."

"Where is she?"

"I don't know." I raise my right fist. "Don't hit me! She's at Corp HQ, Hub Central. She went there an hour ago. I checked out of curiosity," he says by way of explanation.

"Ok," I really don't have a lot of time. "Here's what I want you to do." I want a one-way ticket to Eden. Tonight.

"Can't be done," he says, "tickets to Eden were closed. No explanation."

Tessa, I think. "Find a way."

He looks at me and reconsiders his options. "Ok, it'll cost!"

I let him scan my implanted credit chip and his eyes nearly pop out of his sockets. "It'll take most of that," he warns.

"Just get it done!"

He nods. "Come back in an hour."

I leave without another word. On my way out I bend down and strip a mini-blaster from the waistband of one of the fallen goons. I was unnecessarily harsh with Snug and his men but it was the only way to get his attention. Information peddlers, amongst other things, have no allegiance. I needed him to know that the stakes on this one are high. One wrong word and he will be joining Red Reaper stats.

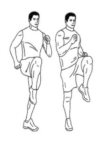

200 high knees

***

Corporate HQ. Not the best place to loiter outside of. I merge with those passing across the street from them, use the vehicles and heavy traffic to disguise my movements. My hood is up. I look out from underneath it gauging activity.

The place is heavily defended. Not that this is something that stops me. I have successfully infiltrated military camps. I know that all the energy goes on the outside. Pierce the defense and get past their protocols and then, working from the inside makes you almost unstoppable.

From the level of activity on the forecourt outside I can see that for them it's business as usual. My guess is that Tessa is not even there any more. A person who blocks flights to Eden out of precaution will have doubled guard security and put the place on alert as a matter of course. I know that this now sounds like I have an ego the size of a planet-sized moon, but I am actually that good. She would have taken every precaution, regardless.

From her perspective she may have bested me in the desert and locked me up at the scientific station to become her guinea pig but she had no way of knowing what kind of resources I could bring to bear.

The fact that everything looked normal argued that she was on the move again. And I knew where she was heading. Dock 17, was about to see more action than it had ever bargained for.

This time, I take the back streets. And I run to get there on time.

**

Docks are incredibly busy places. As the name suggests shuttles come and go all the time, so they have holding areas, for cargo, staging areas for passengers. Sales desks to tickets, stands for all sorts of merchandise imaginable. There are credit stations where you can buy and sell credit chips.

There are minor banks and major lending houses. There are soldiers of fortune waiting to get hired and freelance Regulators who can be had to escort VIPs around the Hub as they conduct their business.

In other words, passing inconspicuous in a Dock is easy, provided you don't start a firefight or get into a face-off with the local law. My guess was that Leonidas, Ellie's uncle, would be coming in with a personal shuttle service. Maybe his own security. A message from the Wired is enough to make anyone paranoid and Ellie's family sounded like this was the kind of thing they took in their stride.

I get there with sweat dripping off me. It's getting to be a thing with me this trip. I take the first elevator shaft I find and go up to the sky restaurants. I need a bird's eye-view and have no recourse to any tech.

Restaurants have a foyer. Robo screeners scan each guest for attire, weapons and then, finally, creditworthiness, in that order. From the order you understand where their priorities lie. Looks are everything. I am not dressed for dining. This means I have just a minute or two before the Robo screener asks me to leave. I don't dwell on the ignominy of not even being able to get a seat at a restaurant. The moment I get to the top I walk over to the glass wall on the far side, overlooking the Dock below and scan it fast.

Crates. Rob workers. Automated tracks. Regulator security. Security. Auto dump tracks. Ships in various stages of parking. Ships rolling out, readying for take-off. Ships coming in. People. Passengers. Security. Robots. Regulators. The images below break up into so many kaleidoscopic fragments, each laden with its own importance.

I scan each one looking for the anomaly. Regulators. Robo guards. Regulators. My eyes stop on a batch of Regulators standing absolutely still. Guns ready. They have their back to an alley created by several towering stacks of aluminium containers. From the 100-floor high observatory I cannot see more than that. The containers hide the passage way their bulks create. But the guards standing still is an anomaly.

Freight is valuable. Buildings. Tracks even - maybe. Ships.

Not alleys or passageways. Unless something is going on inside them.

"Gotcha!" I say to myself. And turn to head back to the nearest elevator just as its doors are closing and a Robo screener is approaching me.

"I am sorry," it says with its flat, modulated voice. "Steel meshed attire is not permitted in the dining area."

"Too bad!" I can't resist saying. I push past it, unbalancing it on purpose. Its whole attention, momentarily, is on regaining its balance and by then I am through a service door and looking down at 100 flights of stairs. Great! This side will get me nearest the Regulator guards I saw from above.

I have the choice of waiting for the elevator to come up and take it down or take one of the others ones and then re-orient myself to get to the Regulators and whatever is going on in the alley on time. I have no choice, really. The stairs it is. I start taking them two at a time, swearing under my breath.

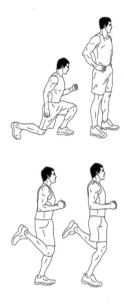

10 reverse lunges
20 butt kicks
10 reverse lunges
20 butt kicks
10 reverse lunges
20 butt kicks
10 reverse lunges
20 butt kicks
10 reverse lunges
20 butt kicks

I come out at the bottom of the restaurant with my now familiar sweaty face. It occurs to me that every time I see Tessa I am almost out of breath. I grin, but there's no humor to it.

Using the cover of tracks and people moving I manage to get near the Regulators unnoticed. I am still a good 50m away from them and hiding behind a stack of what look like armored suitcases. Right now, I would give anything for my own large blaster, but I have to work with what I have. I take out the mini-blaster I liberated from Snug's goon and sprint the other way, circling to get to the alley from the back.

I figure that really it is the action inside I should busy myself with and tackling the Regulator guards would alert Tessa and her cohorts. The other side is mostly blocked by containers placed in a haphazard way. I squeeze past them and suddenly I have a front-row seat to what's unfolding inside.

Ellie is on the ground, holding her cheek. There is a redness there where she's obviously been struck. Raynar is up against one of the containers. His back pressed against it. A mini-blaster aimed at his neck by a Regulator. It seems his past allegiances buy him no favors.

Reed is on his knees. Lips bleeding. He's been roughed up. There are three bodies on the ground. Unmoving. Private security. Clearly not worth the money it cost. There are missing parts of them and the scattered red dust I can see around them tells me all I need to know. Mini-blasters have done their work.

There are two more Regulators there. Weapons drawn. But it's the two people standing at the very center of all that which hold my attention. One is a man I don't know. I assume it is Leonidas Ri, Ellie's uncle. The other one, of course, is Tessa. She's changed into a slick black uniform since I saw her in the desert. I have seen that before. It's the same slick black non-regulation, Regulator uniform that Captain Jackal was wearing in his hologram, when he spoke to us.

In a tight corner, surprise is the biggest weapon. The next best thing is chaos. I step smoothly out of the shadows, bring up the mini-blaster in my hand and turn the head of the Regulator that had been holding Raynar pressed against the container into so much red dust.

The scene explodes into movement. The other two, surprised begin to raise their weapons, eyes looking for targets. They are trying to understand what happened. I give them no chance.

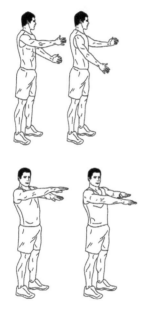

keep arms up throughout

20 scissor chops

10 arm scissors

20 scissor chops

10 arm scissors

20 scissor chops

10 arm scissors

20 scissor chops

10 arm scissors

20 scissor chops

10 arm scissors

You can't fire too many shots in contained situations like this. Chances are you're going to hit a friendly and I have come to like Raynar and feel kinda responsible for Ellie.

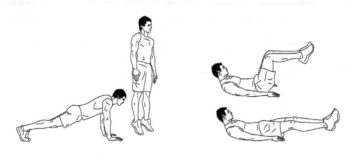

20 basic burpees (no push-ups) + **ONE** crunch kick

A little. So, I shoulder roll to the first one. Kick him in the stomach as I get up.

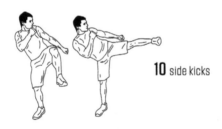

10 side kicks

Follow it up with another kick to the head as he doubles up in pain.

He goes down like he's been poleaxed. I love my boots.

Raynar takes care of the other goon.

"You Ok?" I help Ellie to her feet. She nods.

As the action exploded, Reed darted on hands and knees to one side. Taking himself out of the target zone. Smart.

If Tessa is surprised to see me she doesn't show it.

"We meet again," I say, but there is no mirth in my voice.

"The Red Reaper alive and well," says Tessa and I sense the change in the atmosphere in those around me. The tension in the air. Surprise? Shock? Fear? I really can't tell.

"Looks like Captain Jackal shares your taste in clothes," I say and she brushes it off with a shrug.

I am about to say something profound about justice and revenge but I don't get the chance. A white flash zings just past my head, bounces off the metal wall of a contained behind me. The Regulators left guarding the entrance to this makeshift alley are running towards us. Guns firing.

Tessa takes the opportunity to pull out her own weapon. More flashes from the Regulators, thankfully badly aimed because they're running. Tessa fires. I see everything in slow mo. Her aim is off. She's more rattled than she lets on. She misses me by a good half foot. The Regulators are some distance off.

Leonidas Ri has Ellie in his arms. He whirls her about shielding her unnecessarily with his own body. It's a stupid move. Blasters turn everything into red dust. You can't really shield someone else that way. Reed is huddled against one of the metal walls, about as far away from me as he can get. He's whimpering, his characteristic cool shattered by circumstances.

Raynar is off and moving. He knows he can't tackle Regulators without a weapon, yet he's stupid enough to try. Stupid, stupid, pride. Tessa brings her right arm back in line with me. Her left hand moves to cradle the right. Classic handgun pose. She's providing a steadied firing platform for herself.

I breathe in. Slowly. Deeply. I have always been able to think clearly in a gunfight. I move my body just half a foot, spin sideways. My right foot stretched out. I catch Raynar on the ankle as he tries to run past.

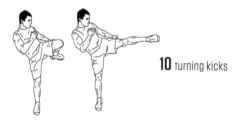

10 turning kicks

He lets out a groan of surprise, loses his balance, arms windmilling, he sprawls. Twin beams of white flash over where his head would have been but a second before.

Tessa's carefully aimed shot misses. The beam goes harmlessly past me. I shoot her first. I take no chances and she's way too close. The mini-blaster in my hand sings. Nanoseconds before her head disappears in a cloud of red dust I register that she looks surprised.

Her death causes confusion. The Regulators running towards us momentarily stumble. They try to process the implication of what they're seeing. I am counting on just that. Human psychology is terribly predictable. I drop to one knee presenting a smaller target. Take aim and fire.

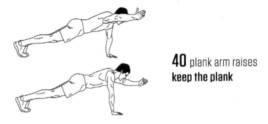

40 plank arm raises
keep the plank

The legs of one of the Regulators disappear. His torso falls face down. The systemic shock already killing him. His comrade knows he's next. He fires off a wild shot missing us all completely. Tries to backtrack and too late seek cover. My next beam takes away his left arm. Then his left leg. He falls and doesn't move.

I catch movement and turn. Leonidas Ri is on his feet pulling Ellie away. "Don't kill us," he implores me.

"Why should I? I risked my life to send you the message through the Wired."

He looks confused.

"The Red Reaper?" Raynar spits out. He's picking himself up. His ego bruised more than his hands and knees.

I shrug. There's nothing to say to this, now.

"You butchered - "

"No one-" I cut him off abruptly and the tone of my voice stops him in his tracks. "I butchered Regulators who wiped out a mining colony using banned weapons. I just didn't stay behind to control the narrative is all I did."

Does he believe me? But then again, why should I lie?

"You could have told us sooner," from Reed. Suddenly everyone's ego is hurt.

"I don't go around advertising my presence. Besides, I'm retired."

"The Galaxy's most famous assassin retired? You're kidding?"

"No, I am not." I try to explain it all to them quickly. "I was on my way to some place else when all this went down. I got sucked into it, just like you."

Maybe they believe me. Maybe not. It doesn't matter. I have a ticket to get and a shuttle to catch. "You'd better get some decent security," I turn to Leonidas. "Xelium production is not something corporations take kindly being messed with. He nods. Places a protective arm around Ellie.

"You lied to us," Raynar appears to take my deceit particularly hard.

"No, not lied. I just never completely told you who I was."

"The Red Reaper?" he's repeating himself. I guess he needs time to process this. They clearly don't make Regulators the way they used to.

"Don't stay here long," I admonish Reed. I turn to go.

"Where are you going?" from Raynar.

"I have as flight to catch. This is where I am supposed to be. You guys should be OK now." I nudge Tessa's headless body with my foot. "This, won't be bothering you anymore."

"Just like that? You're leaving?" Raynar persists.

"What'd you expect? Flowers?"

He frowns.

"Find a better outfit to join next time. Regulators are less and less palatable these days." I say.

I leave without saying any more goodbyes. I find goodbyes ridiculous. Too much sentiment compressed in brief moments that cloud all judgement. On the way out to the far end of passageway, I stop to pick up one more blaster from the downed Regulators. You never know, I think to myself. I am not off this planet just yet.

Chapter 26

In my life I have much to atone for. I did not become an assassin by design but my notoriety rests upon a false premise: Orion. I killed the killers. But those who sent the killers controlled the narrative. I became the patsy.

Admittedly I have used that notoriety to my advantage. Those who might wish to double-cross you, think twice about it if they think they're dealing with a person that wiped out an entire colony. Tessa represented everything I hate about the corporations and their Regulator muscle. Ending her was instinctive. The fact that her death also throws a wrench in the corporation bio-weapons program is a boon.

I tell myself that I would miss none of this. For too long I have had to live with deals and compromises, navigating a delicate balance between those who needed to be killed and those who have the means to order the death of anybody. As an assassin I've always chosen the jobs that came my way. And money has never been the only criterion for me.

Movement snaps me out of my self-indulgent thoughts. I've been walking through the crowd, hood up, head down, the long overgarment covering me, hiding my gait. There is movement all around me, so whatever I picked up out of the corner of my eye has alerted a part of my brain that does not use thoughts, or words.

Surreptitiously I look up. Regulators! Lots of them, at least a dozen, bearing the black patch insignia of Captain Jackal's division. Lovely. I watch them jostle through the crowd, a couple of them coming to within five yards of me. I have both my blasters at the ready.

Hands gripping them tightly in my pockets. But they just storm past, pushing people aside as if they are nothing but obstacles to be navigated through.

I get to Snug's place, check carefully for any outside attention and then I cross the street, into the alley and through his front door. It has been left ajar and that alerts me. I feel more than see the crashing blow coming my way. A massive metal bat swung viciously with both hands by one of Snug's stupid goons.

I duck. Spin. Kick the knee of his front leg.

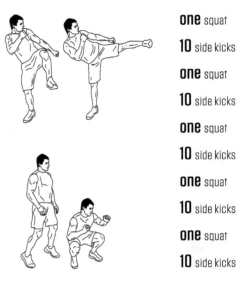

one squat

10 side kicks

one squat

10 side kicks

one squat

10 side kicks

one squat

10 side kicks

one squat

10 side kicks

The metal bat, having completed its swing crashes harmlessly against the wall behind me at the same time as my boot connects with the goon's knee. There is an ugly pop of cartilage tearing and he screams and goes down clutching his knee with both hands.

I step over his writhing body and coolly place the nozzle of the mini-blaster against the forehead of the other goon who has not yet taken in quite what has just happened. "You moved so fast-" he said eyes blinking with shock.

"Snug," I say to the figure cowering behind the counter. "If you don't have my ticket I swear I am going to redecorate this place with your brains."

"I have it." One trembling hand appeared over the counter, holding a digiplaque aloft. How quaint. I haven't seen one of these for a long time, didn't even know they were still in use. Rectangular, holographed. Marked with the itinerary ship's name and holding the record of a passage, paid in full. "I have it," Snug repeats and the hand holding the digiplaque is joined by the top of his head, and then his eyes.

"Stand up," I bark.

He obeys. He seems less than pleased to see me. "I have it," he says again pointlessly.

"Tell your goon to back off," I bark again.

Snug nods and the big, meaty bloke backs off. I watch him go and help his buddy who is still groaning, off the floor. The goon I kicked is limping, badly. You just don't mess with steel mesh boots. He leans on his friend and hobbles away on one leg.

"Me and you," I turn to Snug.

"I didn't know if you'd come back," he says defensively.

"Theresa Fui Draconum is not the kind of person who leaves people alive."

So, that was her full name. Interesting. Even more interesting that Snug knew what it was. I take a note of it and instantly make the connection. So very obvious in retrospect. Story of my life, I think and the thought mellows me. I smile at Snug.

"You've been eavesdropping on Regulator comms," I say to him.

"Lots of chatter. They're bringing reinforcements."

My tight smile makes him back off.

"I never said anything about you. I really didn't!"

I believe him. This place would be a deathtrap for all of us if he had.

"Give me the ticket."

He does. The digiplaque is rectangular in shape. Micron-thin. Made of metal. These things are supposed to be impossible to counterfeit. I assume it's the real thing, but ...

"It's real?"

"Real. Real." Snug volunteers immediately. "Can't get past first scan with a fake one. These things are so hard to get hold of right now."

He's right, they are. But he's also building up the value. The cost.

"Have I got any credit left?" I ask.

"You have a little. But not much."

Ok, at least in this he is honest. A little would have to do. I can get hold of more money when I get to Eden. I place the digiplaque in a pocket.

"Don't think of blabbing," I warn.

He blanches. Shrinks away from me to the very back of the wall behind the counter. I slip back outside.

Everything in my life breaks down into tasks. Tasks are governed by goals. Goals reveal my purpose. I have to get the ship to get to Eden. I need to be in Eden to disappear completely. There I have all the resources required to make the Red Reaper a thing of legend, more fairy tale than real. It is only by disappearing that I can reclaim my life. Finally be free of what I am.

I repeat all this in my head a few times. Just to remind myself of the stakes. I have already burnt through a mountain of credits to get to this point and my detour,

thanks to Ellie and her father's solution to the coming
Xelium shortage, hasn't helped.

My way to the staging area where ship passengers are
processed is marked by Regulator patrols, more than a few of
them of the Jackal's division and the occasional commotion.
The Hub always feels like a pressure cooker about to explode.
There are just too many people in too little a space. Despite
this I manage to almost get to where I need to without
incident. Almost.

"You murdering bastards! Let me go!" The voice is familiar.
And female.

Without drawing attention to myself I raise my head a little,
peer from beneath by hood. Regulators. A group of them, in
4x4 formation. Black insignia at their throats. Great! In their
midst, they are dragging a body, legs flailing. Arms bound
tight. I catch a glimpse of familiar hair, a face. Ellie.
Damn it kid.

I stop dead in my tracks. Just ahead the staging area

beckons. Digiplaque holders get VIP treatment. There is a lounge with dimmed walls to wait. One of the holographic displays overhead announces the flight to Eden is leaving in an hour.

This trip I have had the worst of luck. An hour. I can't draw attention here, so my pivot is gentle. I take care to regulate my step with those around me. I turn around and follow the glimpses of the Regulators ahead long enough to gauge their direction.

Then, melting through the crowd I get to the backstreets and the back alleys and break into a run.

Rounding the first corner I cannonball into a massive bulk of a man carrying something breakable. I know it's breakable because, as you can guess, by the time I pick myself up from having bounced off him, whatever he was carrying lies in broken glass shards all around us.

"Hey!"

"Sorry," I make to take off again and a massive hand wraps itself up around my wrist.

"Hey!" he says again which may be either anger and surprise or he really has a very limited vocabulary. Either way I have no time to find out which it is. I turn on him. He's holding my wrist really tight because he expects me to try and pull away, but I pivot instead on my right leg, my back now moving towards him and my elbow comes down hard on the inside of the arm holding me.

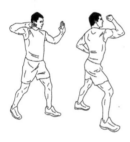

20 upward elbow strikes

He lets out a cry and the grip relaxes enough for me to pull my wrist loose.

"Sorry," I hiss and the cold tip of my blaster touches the base of his neck, exactly at the throat. "Try that again and there'll be songs about you to match the Orion mounds," I hiss.
The reference makes him blanch. He squints at me, actually seeing me for the very first time and then his face blanches.

"Hey," he says softly - clearly he's turned that into a multi-purpose word. I have no time to exchange tips on communication theory. I shove him back and watch him fall, the will to fight clearly gone out of him. And I am off. Running fast. Jumping over every obstacle placed in my path.

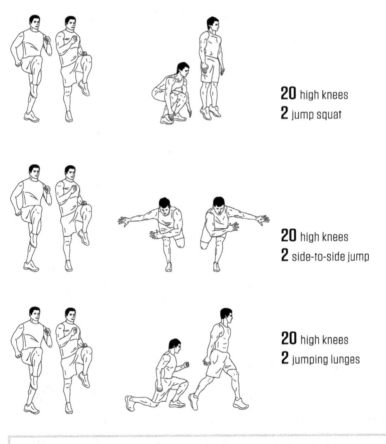

20 high knees
2 jump squat

20 high knees
2 side-to-side jump

20 high knees
2 jumping lunges

catch your breath, rest up to 2 minutes, and repeat the circuit
7 times in total

I catch up with the Regulators about a kilometer away but I am already too late. There are just two left now and Ellie is nowhere in sight. I cut in front of them and they instantly recognize me. They try to bring up weapons but I am already too close for that. Stupid decision on their part, really.

The first one gets my knee. It's a full thrust to the stomach delivered with the entire force of my run. It lifts him off his feet.

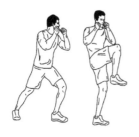

40 knee strikes

The plated armor he is wearing takes most of the blow but enough penetrates to crack the soft bone and cartilage in the sternum. It makes a loud enough sound even for me to hear it and he goes down like he's been poleaxed.

The second fumbles his weapon draw. It snugs in his holster and he panics. I crack his clavicle, breaking the collarbone and immobilizing him.

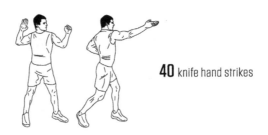

40 knife hand strikes

He lets out a howl and falls to his knees, arm dangling uselessly to the side.

"Where's Ellie?" I ask.

He looks perplexed.

"Ellie, the girl you had. Where is she?"

"Captain Jackal," he says. "He wants to see her. We're taking her to him."

There's something in his voice that suggests I should be afraid of that but I don't know enough to be afraid.

"Where?"

"Huh?" he's playing dumb. I pistol whip him across the face breaking his nose and badly lacerating the skin.

"Where is Captain Jackal," I say.

He looks at me through eyes, now red with blood. "RIM Corp," he whispers, "We are taking her to our HQ."

My next blow knocks him unconscious.

RIM Corp. Damn! I need to buy myself some time. I need to buy Ellie some time. I search the two Regulator bodies. One of them is carrying a transmitter. I am hoping it's on the correct frequency because I only have this shot.

"Red Reaper, calling Captain Jackal. Red Reaper calling Captain Jackal. Over."

Silence . Then, just as I had given up on receiving a reply, I hear the crackle of an incoming voice: "Red Reaper? Really?"

"In the flesh,"

"Well, well," the glee gives it away. Captain Jackal can barely hide his emotion. "That really you?"

"Tessa thought so," I say.

As expected he pauses, processing this. When he speaks next he sounds perplexed. "My sister? Tess?"

"Your late sister," I correct.

"You're lying!"

Now I am the one who's confused. I assumed Ellie and the others were picked up at Dock 17, with all those bodies surrounding them. Clearly this is not the case. I tell myself to solve this one later. Now I need Captain Jackal to listen. "Check out Dock 17 - DNA scan. You'll find some interesting smears amongst the red dust piles.

"No!"

"Her Chimera-creating days are over."

"You're going to pay for this!"

"Fui Draconum," I say, "really?"

"It's an old family name."

"Clearly. And not many people speak Latin anymore." The Classics are not of much use in space.

"I will kill you."

"Maybe. You still have the girl?"

"Why?"

"As long as you have her and she's in one piece I am prepared to bargain for her."

"What do you offer?"

"My life, for hers. In one hour."

"Deal!"

Rarely have I heard so much pain, death and venom in a voice, distilled into a single word. Maybe our good Captain truly loved his sister. A little Chimera-producing team. I crash the transmitter underfoot. These things can be tracked.

I am running once more. Just as fast as before.

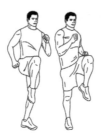

200 high knees

I know what I've done. I've bought Ellie some time. As long as Captain Jackal thinks he may have to give me proof of life before I hand myself over he will keep her alive and intact. Of course, I have no intention of giving myself up.

Chapter 27

I find myself back where I started, staring at the alleyway hiding Snug's shop. I cross the road realizing I am drenched in sweat again. This time the door is locked. I palm the bio-reader and there is a short delay before the door swings open.

When I enter, cautiously, the two goons have been replaced by four new ones. These ones are dressed in black. They look slicker. And they have theirs guns out.

"You're back!"

I can't quite read Snug's voice this time.

"Happy to see me?" I ask, ignoring the goons and the guns.

"Your ship is leaving in less than 30 minutes. Why are you not there?"

"Pressing business," I say. I bring out the digiplaque. "I need you to take this back,"

"What?" he looks at me like I am crazy. The four goons around me shuffle taking a few steps back, uncertain. Their guns are still pointing at me.

"And I want a few supplies in return, instead." I give him my list.

"You're crazy."

"Make it happen," I say.

"You think you're in a position to bargain?" He dares to put a little sneer in his voice. It's a mistake. People, I think, just keep making mistakes around me.

I whip out a hand faster than any of them can react. Grab Snug by the throat and pull him forward so that his face hits the counter in front of him. I know. Classic undercover cop or underdog brutality maneuver. It is. But it also works. And because it's such a cliche everyone is ready to believe it.

My other hand is holding the mini-blaster to his face.

"Don't! Please don't!" he whimpers.

"I only have to twitch and your head will be dust," I say.

"Please."

The goons are frozen in their tracks. Uncertain what to do.

"Tell them to drop their guns and stand back," I say. Snug does just that. "Good. Now tell them to help put the stuff on the list together." I try not to smile as Snug complies and they jump to help.

In my head I am busy joining dots. Captain Jackal's black insignia-ed thugs did not pick up Ellie at Dock 17. If they had they'd have known already about Tessa's unfortunate mishap with my blaster. This means that they'd either been tipped off and picked her up on the way or they just got lucky and came across her and the others. If it's A I've been betrayed. Maybe. If it's B the others are dead. No one has any real use for them and they know too much.

Corporations cannot let their experimentation with bio-weapons or their use of banned weapons get out. The only way to ensure it doesn't is to wipe out every trace of everyone who might know something. In a moment of deja vu I see myself wading through a future marked by training swirls of red dust. I shake it off.

"Who did you talk to Snug?" I ask as the goons are busy with the assembly of my new shopping list.

"No one. I haven't left my property," he says like he's talking to an idiot.

"Why did Captain Jackal tell me he spoke to you then?" I am fishing.

He blanches just a little. Too little for me to be 100% sure, and holds his ground. "Captain who?"

"Fui Draconum," I say, "Tessa's brother, remember? Or should I say the surviving sibling of the Fui Draconum family?"

My gambit pays off, he momentarily loses it. His eyes blink rapidly. He licks his lips. "You killed her? You killed Theresa Fui Draconum?" he asks using her full name.

"Come clean you louse or I shall be adding you to my confirmed body count," I say. I don't really know if there is a confirmed body count. Being the bogeyman of the galaxy means they pin all sorts of stuff on you as an excuse for their own failures or simply because you're a convenient target.

Corps take out a container ship who's captain has been skimming a little off the side? It was the Red Reaper. Some corporate vendetta comes to a messy end, again, my name comes up. And should government lackeys decide to get mixed up in some internal 'house clearing', yep, you can bet it's going to be pinned on me.

As a matter of fact I think that if we actually track all the kills attributed to me and work back on the timeline it will be proved that I can miraculously be in several places at the exact same time. Snug, I know, is weighing all he knows and has heard about me in this moment.

I take a half step towards him.

"Please!" he begs cowering, "don't kill me!" On cue, a goon appears, then another.

"Back to work you." I bark at them.

They don't listen. The first one takes a step towards me. Misguided loyalty to his new boss makes him stupid. That plus ignorance of who I really am. What I am capable of. It's a mistake.

I duck under the first goon's overswing. Where does he even find these people?

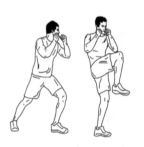
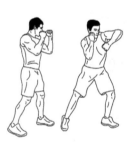

8 knee strikes - right knee

10 elbow strikes - right elbow

8 knee strikes - left knee

10 elbow strikes - left elbow

8 knee strikes - right knee

10 elbow strikes - right elbow

8 knee strikes - left knee

10 elbow strikes - left elbow

8 knee strikes - right knee

10 elbow strikes - right elbow

8 knee strikes - left knee

10 elbow strikes - left elbow

catch your breath, rest up to 2 minutes, and repeat the circuit
3 times in total

I kick him twice, left knee, right knee, then knee him in the stomach as he falls and elbow-strike him in the face. Close-quarters combat is all about applying the right amount of force on joints.

The second is behind me before the first one's unconscious body completely collapses on the floor and then I have to half spin to avoid his grip, body moving as a weapon. I slam into him with my back, unbalancing him.

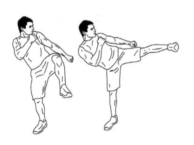
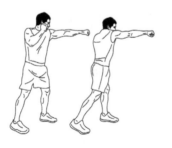

10 side kicks - left leg

20 punches

- switch sides -

10 side kicks - right leg

20 punches

- switch sides -

10 side kicks - left leg

20 punches

- switch sides -

10 side kicks - left leg

20 punches

catch your breath, rest up to 2 minutes, and repeat the circuit
3 times in total

He goes down like an empty sack.

"You were saying," I turn to Snug. Two more goons appear, they see their crumpled comrades on the floor. Look at me.

"Get to work," I repeat and this time they disappear to the backroom they came from. I turn to Snug.

"Please! I'm sorry!"

"What did you do?"

"I told Captain Michail Fui Draconum. I told him where to find the girl and her uncle. Forgive me!"

"Why?"

"I thought you'd be on your way. On the shuttle, on your way to Eden. I didn't sell out your friends. Just the girl and her uncle."

Again: "Why?"

"There's a reward. Lots of credits. Even more than they're paying for you."

"Really?"

"Yes! I'm sorry! It was a mistake!"

As I am contemplating what to do with him the two goons from the back come back. They each have a massive leather bag filled with goodies. I take the bags from them, ask them to back against the far wall. Snug is expecting retribution.

"You betrayed me," I start and he cringes further. "You know much about the Fui Draconum family. How?"

"I've done business with them. Please!" he begs.

"What sort of business?"

"Information. I hear a lot here, at the Hub. They wanted me to be on the lookout for some things. Mentions, rumors, that kind of thing."

"What exactly?"

"Nothing important. Miner stuff. I could never understand their fascination with it."

"Miners?"

"Oh, you know. They wanted scraps of information, anything I could find about Orion families. Then maybe see if I hear something about specific people."

A lot of threads come back to Orion. I wondered ... a thought begins to form at the very back of my mind.

"Betray me again-"

"Technically I didn't-" he begins, which is true but I am not in the mood for semantics.

"Do you want to die?" The goons, just then, remember their task. Take a step forward. I raise an arm their way, finger extended towards the ceiling in admonition. They think better of it and fall back. "Good boys," I say.

"Please," Snug begs.

"No more information sharing from you for today," I say, I stress my words.

Snug looks up. He's not stupid. "Just today?"

"Yup."

"Ok. I swear."

I shoulder the bags and make my way out. It's a little darker now outside. The Hub sun is beginning to set. Perfect. I have a rendezvous with a jackal to keep.

Chapter 28

I am outside and it's getting dark. The alley is deserted but, humping two bags over my shoulder I am extra careful. I hear a noise at the very far end where the shadows bleed into deep darkness.

The Hub is not the kind of place where you want to take your chances when the deck is not stacked for you. I have a brief vision of Regulators with dark insignia on their lapels or maybe the Hub's special brand of muggers.

I take off, the load of the bags weighing heavy on me and my boots striking the Hub surface beneath me with exaggerated force. Whatever was in that alley is soon left behind.

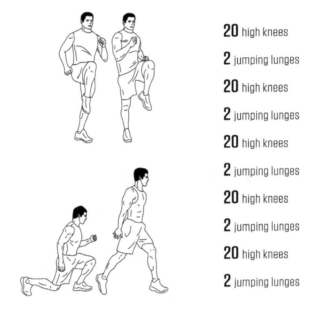

20 high knees

2 jumping lunges

20 high knees

2 jumping lunges

20 high knees

2 jumping lunges

20 high knees

2 jumping lunges

20 high knees

2 jumping lunges

catch your breath, rest up to 2 minutes, and repeat the circuit
3 times in total

Running while being weighed down is never easy. I take care to pick my route so I don't run into a crowd. I have the sense that I am being followed but think to myself that this is me being paranoid. If it was Regulators I'd have been picked up already and if it was muggers, well …

I run.

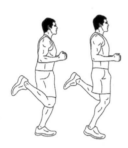

100 butt kicks

Out of breath and within reach of RIM Corp, Regulators HQ in the Hub. I used the time I was running to clear my head and formulate a plan. The easiest, I know, is never the best.

I could go in all guns ablaze. Create so much red dust that there'll be more tales told about me, but that's not really my style. There are Regulators in there who don't deserve that. So here I am, hiding behind the last available cover, watching RIM Corp carefully through a pair of augmented reality binoculars that give me all sorts of telemetrics.

I think to myself that this must be partially what Reed felt like all the time. The thought of the hacker adds to my sense of sadness and drip-feeds my anger. I notice that I've used the past tense yet I have no evidence that he is, indeed, dead. The thought momentarily distracts me. Never a good thing to happen in the Hub.

"Daydreaming?" Spoken softly, off to my right and I get to my feet. Fast. My right hand is already reaching for my blaster when I recognize the voice through the whispered undertones.

"Raynar?"

The Regulator steps out from behind cover. Reed on his heels. I feel like hugging them both but the gesture would be out of place right now and I have not forgotten what I am here to do.

"Missed us?" asks the Regulator. He sounds matter-of-fact but I sense there is anger in his voice.

"What happened?" I ask.

"The Jackal happened," he says. "We were clear of the Docks, Ellie and her uncle going home. Reed and thinking of getting somewhere we could spend a day or two figuring out what to do next. Jackals men intercepted Ellie, killed her uncle and his hired muscle. Took the girl prisoner. Reed here intercepted messages from across the intranet."

I nodded. His words filled in all the blanks. "How did you find me?" I ask.

"Oh, that was Reed," says Raynar.

I look over to Reed and the hacker looks sheepish. Then: "I put a tracer on you. Just in case." he says at last. Looks down.

"You tagged me?" I am trying to remember how it could have happened.

"Back at Dock 17," he says seeing me frowning. He understands I am thinking back. "All that melee with Tessa and those goons in black. I thought that if you took off and we needed you we had no way of finding you. Plus ..." he pauses and shuffles his feet a little, looking at the ground. "All that Red Reaper stuff. There's a huge reward out for you. I thought it wouldn't hurt knowing where you are." He lifts his head to look at me now.

My reputation is a burden as well as a boon. I understand why he did what he did. "Where? Where's the tag?" He does that thing he does behind his eyes. The pupils momentarily unfocus and then, I feel the slightest buzz at the back of my neck. Just under the hairline. Clever. Hackers.

"It's off," he says.

I rub my hand at the hairline and it comes away with the thinnest of skin scales. Almost entirely transparent. No wonder I never felt it.

"Why are you here?" More to the point.

"We're here to help," from Raynar.

"Yeah, no way you're doing this alone," confirms Reed.

In my life, most times, I've operated alone. Sure I make and use friends and allies here and there but really, because they usually die, I prefer to work alone. That way the nightmares I have late at night are not populated with people I liked.

"No way," I say and mean it. They have no idea what they're getting into.

"Yes way," says Raynar. Childish retort really. I shrug. Begin to turn away. I know I need to get rid of them both. "What's your plan anyway?"

I turn back to look at him. He's stands cocky, hands on hips. He knows now that he can't really take me even if he tried his hardest but still. "I'm going to create a diversion. Infiltrate it and then clear the rooms, one by one until I find Ellie and free her," I say. It sounds crazy, even to me, but I haven't really had a lot of time to come up with a plan and now I am just playing for time.

"That's insane!" says Reed. "How long do you think you'll last in there?"

He has a point but then again they don't quite know everything about me. I have survived some pretty tough odds in my life.

"If three of us worked it, wouldn't it be easier? Improve the odds of getting Ellie out alive?" asks Raynar. It's a reasonable question and I cannot fault the logic of his asking. While I was running I thought of a plan, a couple actually. My brain used the time to clear out its thinking. What I said to Raynar and Reed was correct. It is one of the plans that occurred to me, but only one of them.

It occurs to me, as I'm about to open my mouth, that I may be handing out death sentences. I pause. Mouth open.

"Is a sound going to come out some time?" Raynar asks. His sense of humor is insufferable at times.

"Well?" even Reed is impatient.

Why do people rush in to die but fail to apply the same haste in living a life? The thought has preoccupied me before. I have no answer to it. Not yet.

"There may be a way," I say. "We might be able to pull something off without killing anyone or dying ourselves."

"That would be a trick worthy of the Red Reaper," Raynar says.

"It will take all of us. And a lot of running and climbing." I say.

"We can do it," says Reed. He really doesn't know what he is letting himself in for.

I begin detailing my plan. Reed is the first one to understand it. He pulls up a schematic from a Hub databank. It shows the RIM Corp from the top down, in 3D. We begin to carve out our roles in this, look at each part we have to play in detailed, think of alternative scenarios.

Ping. Time's up. I know that sound.

"Well, are you there?" The Jackal's voice is all choked up with barely suppressed rage. We momentarily all look at the comms device at my waist and then we all silently nod.

We are on!

I raise the device to my lips and answer: "I am here. The girl?"

"Let me see you." the Jackal has a sense of humor then.

"Not a chance. You think I am stupid?"

"You killed my sister. That was a really stupid decision."

"Your sister had it coming. Besides, I saved her first." I don't expect the Jackal to understand this. But he doesn't have to. All I need to do is keep him talking long enough for Reed to work his magic.

On cue. Reed and Raynar take off. They run hunched over. Each holding some of the toys I got from Snug's little toy shop. Telemetry beacons, 3D projectors, some really advanced satellite imaging stuff. They are busy running like hell, setting up an electronic perimeter around RIM Corp as they run. It's going to be funny. I don't think a Regulator HQ has ever been under siege before. This one is going to be one for the history books.

I am counting on the Jackal to do two things: First live up to his name and try and hunt me down quickly and take me alive. And second, double-cross me which means that Ellie is not anywhere easy for me to get to.

RIM Corp follows standard Regulator protocols. It is offices and admin on the outer layer, followed by training suites, living quarters and, finally, in the innermost layer. Holding cells.

"Are you coming in or not?" the Jackal's voice comes in again. Tense. Angry.

"Yeah," I am.

I hear the first siren going off. Reed and Raynar must have now completed putting all the gear in place. On the far side of the RIM Corp building. The side I cannot see because it is furthest away from me I see flares going off and what looks like smoke. It started.

"You're dead!" the Jackal hisses through the comms link and then the device goes dead.

I use the time to run as fast as possible to the far corner of the RIM Corp building.

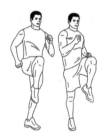

200 high knees

Normally it would be covered by sophisticated electronic surveillance but the equipment I bought from Snug are designed to piggyback on current electronic networks. The AI system governing them sets up a parallel echo that mirrors what is going on around a specific perimeter but then scrubs it clean of intruder data.

The RIM Corp would be hardened against something like this, of course. But I am counting on them not knowing quite the level of sophistication I have brought to bear plus Reed.

Reed, actually, in my revised plan, became the ace up my sleeve.

AI systems are not as smart as most people think they are. They have heuristics that guide them and there is a learning algorithm at their core that helps them adapt to their environment. But they still need to learn new things every time and when time and data are not on their side, they can actually be pretty dumb. But they are fast.

With Reed guiding it the system would receive training data right from the second we deployed it. Plus, Reed would fine tune the parameters. Right now, as Raynar, Reed and I ran to the RIM Corp building and started climbing up one of the steep walls that had no windows, the system rendered us invisible. All the surveillance equipment, looking down at us, were being overridden and told to scrub us from their memory.

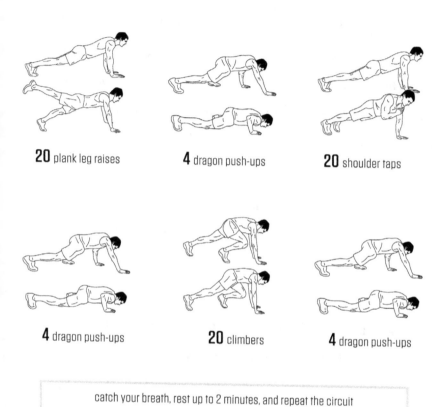

20 plank leg raises   4 dragon push-ups   20 shoulder taps

4 dragon push-ups   20 climbers   4 dragon push-ups

catch your breath, rest up to 2 minutes, and repeat the circuit
3 times in total

To confuse the system further the AI would be throwing up
false flags. Setting off perimeter alarms in areas we were
nowhere near.

Carrying some extra equipment still the climb up a steep wall is not easy. I use grapplers in feet and hands, old-school ninja style. There is no electronic signature and because there is no powerpack either I can guarantee they will not run out and strand me.

I work up quite the sweat and then Reed's voice crackles in the intercom in my ear: "Ellie's on the twelfth floor, not the basement," he says.

My guess is that he's been interrogating the smart system that runs the building. I do not ask how he knows or if he's sure. I take it that if he says so, he is sure. "Ok," I say. I keep on climbing.

I break through a skylight window on the twelfth using a heat charge to melt a hole in the glass. It's efficient, quiet and fast.

"I am going to find you," the Jackal's voice comes through the comms device on my belt. I dial down the sound. Last thing I want is to have him give my position away when I am inside.

"I thought I was dead," I say deadpan. I want to enrage him further.

"We shall find you," he yells back. This time I kill the comms. He's angry which means he's not thinking clearly.

"Reed, Raynar, you guys OK?" I whisper.

Reeds voice comes in first: "Peachy."

Then Raynar: "They can't spot us and we're not out in the open. We're cool."

Relieved I push on.

Inside the building I stop to get my bearings. Reed's schematics that showed me the layout come to mind. There are strobes flashing ahead and the building is partially in darkness inside. My guess is this is their lockdown mode. There will be cameras everywhere but thanks to Reed and Snug's clever toys I am invisible to them.

I run down a corridor, find a door, drop half a floor on a flight of steps and then find another corridor to get through.

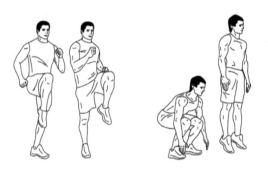

40 high knees and then **2** jump squats

By the time I find where Ellie is being kept I am out of breath. A semi-permanent condition for me this run, I think to myself.

The room she's in is old-style on purpose. Door with heavy lock. No electronic access. The claxons calling emergency in some other part, deep inside the building have drawn everyone else away. Reed's work is genius.

I give the door a few heavy kicks

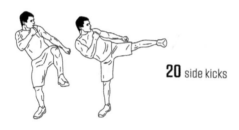

20 side kicks

- and watch the lock buckle. The door swings open with a thud, against the wall. Ellie's inside, curled into a tight ball against the far wall. Even in the low-level lighting of the room I can see the bruises on her face.

"Sef!" she looks up, surprise showing on her face.

"Yeah, I know. I didn't expect to be here either." I tell her. I help her up. She grimaces. "Can you run?"

"Well enough."

"OK, then. Let's go." To the device in my ear I murmur: "Reed, we're heading back. Can you make sure Ellie doesn't show?"

"Got it." Reed is in working mode. His words sparse. Ellie will be scrubbed from all devices just like we are.

We run like mad.

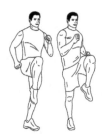

60 high knees

I have my blaster out but we don't meet anyone else. It makes me wonder at just the quality of the cyberdiversions thrown up by the equipment Snug supplied and the scenarios being boosted by Reed and Raynar. We get to the melted window without having to kill anyone.

The climb down is harder. I am supporting Ellie this time and she's heavier than she looks. I am glad for the strength training I've done in the past.

"Once we hit the ground we shall have to sprint to the perimeter. Then arrange to meet up with Raynar and Reed."

"They're here?" Ellie looks up. Despite whatever pain she's in, she seems in good spirits.

I nod. Notice how she lets a smile flit across her face.

We sprint to the perimeter and then crawl the last few hundred yards to the very edge of the cyberprotection offered to us.

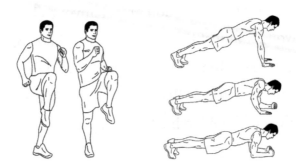

40 high knees and then **10** up and down planks

We both get under cover. When we can both safely look back at the RIM Corp building we see the magnitude of the cyber attack and I then realize just why the building was so empty inside.

There are groups of armed men running in several directions outside. Plumes of smoke and flashing lights are coming from several points of the massive building itself. Internal systems and false alarms. System malfunctions and false readings. RIM Corp were just never ready for that.

I wonder whether I should send one last message to the Jackal but I hear steps, just behind us and turn. Reed is coming towards us, face flushed with sweat. "Their comms are down too," he gasps, "can you believe it? The poor souls are isolated. Completely."

He waits for Raynar to join us before he explains what he's done. The heavy duty AI of the system I brought broke internal encryptions and overwrote all attack and defense algorithms. The RIM Corp building, in effect, started fighting with itself. It still is. "It'll take them hours to sort this stuff out. By then we shall have long gone."

"And Ellie?" I ask.

"Well," Reed says, "The building reports her down in one of the heavy security holding cells in the basement. One that's destined to blow up as a gas main adjacent to it explodes."

It is almost an anticlimax. We see Raynar and Ellie to a launch pad. Quick tickets out of here are purchased.

It feels easy. Too easy but I know that's only in retrospect.
"Where will you go?" I ask.

"My uncle's house. Look for my dad."

"We'll make sure she gets there safely." says Raynar. He puts
out a hand. I take it. "You?"

"I shall go too. Shortly." I say. I am lying. I have a few loose
ends to tie up first.

They both nod.

"Shall we see you again?" from Reed.

"Doubt it. You shouldn't even have seen me the first time."
He and Raynar exchange smiles.

I hang about long enough to make sure that they make it
safely onboard and their flight takes off. I then leave, melting
through back streets and dark alleys. Taking the longest
route from the launch pad back to Hub Central.

Running so as not to use transport and avoiding meeting people whenever I can.

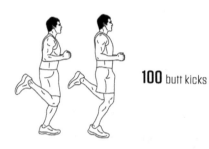

100 butt kicks

There is something still left for me to do. Before I go.

Chapter 29

Alone. At last. Without Reed and Raynar I am aware that I have zero margin for mistakes. I am used to that. I pause to catch my breath and take stock. I am in a back street, poorly lit because no one bothers lighting up back streets.

I have two blasters. A few credits. No ticket out of here and an identity that has now been somewhat compromised. The reward on me is still out there. Skipping out with Raynar, Reed and Ellie, even had I been able to get a new ticket would have put them all at risk.

So, here I am. Doing the right thing, though few would ever consider that this is a prime directive the Red Reaper is driven by. Nevertheless. I know I have to deal with Snug and there is the question of the Jackal still bothering me. But I have more pressing problems to deal with. The lack of credits, right now, is making everything really difficult.

Having recovered I head out again, walking this time. I put my hood up and my head down and I do my best to merge with the crowd. It's a good two clicks to the place I need to and now, time is all on my side.

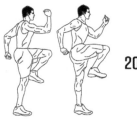

200 march steps

When I get there I scope the streets. Apart from the usual traffic and crowds the area outside is really light on Regulators. I know, of course, that cameras are everywhere and there are drones overhead and by now, what we did at RIM Corp will have stirred things up sufficiently for there to be a major alert out for me.

I wait until there is a break in the traffic and cross over to the other side of the street. My target is a bar at the very end and I use the time it takes to get there to scan everything for suspicious activity. There really is nothing. It surprises me a little.

One last, surreptitious look around and I slip in, pushing past the narrow door, through the full body scanner. It picks up the blasters and beeps and I am instantly surrounded by men in exoskeletons. Weapons in hand and server-assisted muscles at the ready.

"Gents," I raise my arms slowly. "Just two blasters for personal protection," I say. I know the protocol. I have been here before. "I am here to talk business with Cyrus." They pat me down roughly. Strong hands lift my blasters away. One of them throws back my hood. They recognize me instantly, which is not good. My guess on a major alert being out is correct, it seems. It will complicate things. "Cyrus knows me," I add.

They all take a step back. I watch as one of them brings a hand up to his ear. Murmurs something I do not quite catch. Then he turns to the others. "Let him go," he says gruffly. They back off even further. Great. I shrug, readjusting my overcoat.

"Cyrus?" I ask. One of them points with his chin towards the interior behind me.

I leave them behind. Walk in. It's dark. It's noisy. Strobe lights from the stage where some snake-eating act is in progress. I keep walking, past groups, noisy and half-drunk. Couples. Loners. More couples. This is normal Hub bar crowd.

Cyrus is at the far end. Sitting in a darkened corner. Alone. There are two minders off to one side, noticeable by their sheer bulk and the fact that unlike everybody else around us, they do not sway to the beat of the music. I make my way to him and sit down.

"Sef," he acknowledges me. I nod. I've done business with Cyrus before. He's not an entirely trustworthy type of guy but overall he will do what we agree which is all I want now.

"I need a job Cyrus. Is there some work I could do?" Really, I need credits and this is probably the easiest way for me to get some.

"I thought you retired," he says.

I can't tell if he's joking. "Working on it."

"There may be something there for you to do. But it's tricky."

"Then it's costly," I say. I have always been picky about the jobs I take on. Despite what most people think about me I have never been your standard assassin-for-hire. I do need credits right now however and Cyrus has always been a man in need of someone with my special set of skills.

"It always is with you." He leans forward and begins in his own, weird way to explain what it is he needs. Cyrus never speaks straight. There is always a tale he feels he needs to tell or some kind of point he needs to make. I listen as he tells me some weird tale trying to make sure I don't miss the salient points.

We are interrupted by a goon bringing us drinks.

"Not when I am working," I say but Cyrus brushes my objections away. "It's been a long time Sef," he says, "A drink to seal the deal," he raises his glass. I raise mine. We drink almost in unison. It's some sort of local Hub brew. I can taste the afterburn as it goes down.

"So, this job-" I begin. He's looking at me strangely. Or at least I think he is. His eyes appear to be glowing. He blinks and it's like lightbulbs going on and off. I rub my eyes.

"You OK Sef?" He asks.

"Yeah, just tired a bit. All that running." My eyes itch. I find it almost hard to breathe. I get up but there is no strength left in my legs. I find myself looking at the ceiling, strobe lights bouncing off it. Then it goes dark.

I force my eyes open and it takes everything I have to open them just a slit. There are giant shapes looming over me.

Thick voices coming from a long way away. I realize that whatever drug my glass contained slows down processing power in my brain as well as paralyzes the muscles. I am finding it really hard to breathe.

"He's alive," says a voice and I recognize it instantly but the name of its owner escapes me. My drugged brain struggles to make connections.

"As promised. Sef, delivered."

"A call sign for Sanguine Executioner Functional - S.E.F. - The Red Reaper."

"Ah, I didn't know. My reward?"

"As promised," says the voice and the name of its owner comes to me just as the blurry shapes above me loom closer and one of them resolves into the sharp, angular features of Captain Michail Fui Draconum, a.k.a. The Jackal.

***

Red dust everywhere. The worst nightmares always start with swirling red dust. Bodies of ordinary people. Loved ones. Family. Friends. Strangers. Reduced to so much nothingness. It hurts. So much death hurts the senses.

The nightmare strobes like an old movie. I see flashes of Regulators ambushed by me. It always feels like it's not really me. I see the person I will become acting now out of rage. Mad, mad eyes and frothy spittle flying through gritted teeth.

The blasters sing their song and the Regulators, surprised, disappear. Empty suits and burnt visors the only trophy left behind.

The person in the vision lifts the suits. Piles some of them high. Arranges others in special lines or circles. Burns letters onto their chest plates.

Heaving hard as the figure runs.

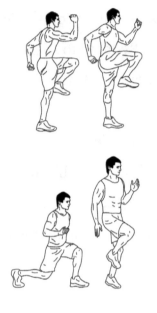

20 march steps

6 lunge step-ups

20 march steps

6 lunge step-ups

20 march steps

6 lunge step-ups

20 march steps

6 lunge step-ups

20 march steps

6 lunge step-ups

In the nightmare the red dust breathed in, is cloying. It makes every step harder, every breath heavier. The whole colony turned to red dust. Regulators wiping out people like life means nothing. Dying themselves, in return, surprised by the person they will come to fear and hate most in the future.

The nightmare suddenly shifts. The scene jumps without explanation into space. Disjointed memories. Some kind of crazy unarmed fight on a ship. Dead bodies lying around on a bridge. Regulator uniforms with blood seeping out.

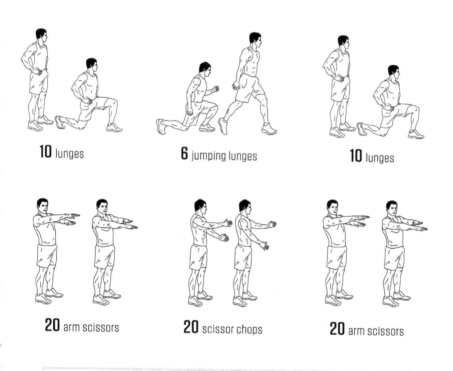

10 lunges   **6** jumping lunges   **10** lunges

20 arm scissors   **20** scissor chops   **20** arm scissors

catch your breath, rest up to 2 minutes, and repeat the circuit
7 times in total

Hands dance at the command controls. Whole banks of outlawed weapons activated. The ships that came with this one. Its comrades in genocide become spectacular starballs in space. Orion below stands empty. A mining colony that reached too far. Sought to unbalance the status quo. Quelled. With no one left to tell the tale. No one. Space is a silent witness.

The nightmare always ends the same way. The turning point in a lifeline. The moment a trained assassin became a legend blamed for something he never did. Taking only jobs that targeted Corps. Funny. Orion had been a Corps op from start to finish. The hit on the miner leader. The Regulators coming next was simply an escalation. Red dust sealed the deal. It also made The Red Reaper.

It made ... me.

Chapter 30

Head hurts. Eyes itch. I am dehydrated. In pain. There are wires coming out of my body. I can't move much. My feet and hands are secured. The room I am in is white. There is a hum somewhere and I am, I guess, on a ship.

Not good. Cyrus sold me out. Bad move.

"Good. You're awake," says a cheerful voice to my right. I turn to look at its owner. A thin guy dressed in white.

"Captain Jackal will be pleased."

Jackal? I think to myself. Do even his own men call him that?

"Can I have some water?" I ask. My tongue feels like dried paper.

"Ah, yeah. The drug they gave you dehydrated you." He does something to one of the consoles in front of him and a robotic arm whirrs by my head. I angle my head to look at it.

"Don't worry," he tells me, "it'll rehydrate you."

The arm stretches out, a scanner reading me. Then it edges closer and a thin needle attached to a tube moves towards me. I stiffen. The cold metal tip touches my neck and there is a painful jab. I say nothing. I see a colorless fluid being pumped in through the tube.

"Fastest way to do this," he says to me by way of explanation. I think to myself that I could easily contest that. A tumbler in my hands would do just the trick but somehow I don't think he really appreciates humor.

I watch him as he goes to the far wall and speaks into a
comm there. Jackal, I guess will be paying me a visit shortly.
I mentally prepare and look around the room. The tube
feeding me liquid through the needle at my neck is beginning
to work. I feel less dehydrated and able to think clearly.

The place is a lab. I can see that now. Neatly folded robotic
arms everywhere. I am strapped down on a gurney.
There are clear tubes in neat rows that I associate with
DNA sequencing. I have seen rooms like that before, one
in particular actually. On the Ghost Ship we boarded I
remember the room with the blood-stained gurneys, the one
that wasn't mentioned in the ship manifest. I realize I may be
in a pickle here and I am angry, really really angry at myself.

I got caught like a rookie because I let my guard down. I
underestimated the resources of the Jackal and the Hub
Regulators. The quiet street scene outside Cyrus' joint,
"too quiet". Clichés! I hate clichés. Worse than that, I hate
becoming them. I test my restraints but they've done their
homework. They have me tied down good.

While waiting for things to unfold I take myself mentally to a serene, quiet place. On Eden I have bought a house. I have a new identity. Credits enough to last me a lifetime. I will wake up every day and go for a run by the sea. Do push ups and pull ups afterwards. Catch up with distant news and watch the latest holovid on the streaming channels.

In my mind, I am running barefoot, on sand next to the morning surf and the sun is really hot on my bare torso. I lift my knees up as I run and pump my arms harder to go faster and the salty air feels fresh on my face. I feel freer and happier than I have ever been in my life...

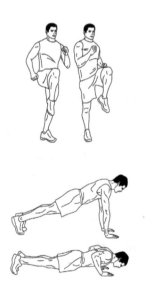

20 high knees
one push-up
20 high knees
one push-up
20 high knees
one push-up
20 high knees
one push-up
20 high knees
one push-up
20 high knees
one push-up

My lungs begin to heave and burn from the effort but I do not let up. I blink rapidly to clear the stinging sweat from my eyes and I take pleasure in this moment where the physical effort of running makes me feel glad to be alive.

"He's awake and lucid," there's a slap on my face. Then another. The voice of the man in white is directly above me and he is slapping me to open my eyes. I am back in the lab, tethered to a gurney and totally helpless. My guess now is he's a Lab Tech.

"Hello," I manage and he slaps me again, a little harder and totally unnecessarily.

"Not so cocky now, are we?" smiles the Jackal. He too looms above me and for the first time, in this very clear light I notice the familial resemblance to Tessa. "You are our very special guest here Sef or-" he pauses for effect, "should I call you Red Reaper?"

"Let me guess," I say, "predictability runs in your family." The grin freezes on his face. I press on, "Dear dead sis Tess paused for effect like that too when she worked it out."

He leans forward and slaps me. In retrospect the Lab Tech in white was gentle like a lamb. "Mention her again," he dares me. He's like a child really. Easy to goad. If it weren't for his special brand of viciousness that allowed him to do the worst things you can imagine he'd never had got as far up the Corps ranks of mercenaries as he has.

"Tess?" I enquire and this time he backhands me. It hurts. I taste the faint, metallic taste of blood in my mouth. "I am tied up a little." I say, "afraid of a fair fight?" Another backhand rewards me with pain. My eyes water with the sting of it.

"I can take you apart here, bit by bit," he says, "we have tech that will keep you alive, awake, lucid while we dismember you. You can get to watch yourself diminish bit by tiny bit."

"What? No holovids to entertain you here?" Another backhand. Harder than before. I think the skin above my cheekbone may have cracked open but I am too numb to feel anything.

"Keep on joking killer. Go ahead. But no one knows you are here. No one knows the fabled Red Reaper got caught in our little trap, like a rookie."

"Trap?"

"Who do you think upped the reward ten-fold?"

"Oh. Right. Greed. Yeah. It's a powerful motivator. But people know I am here-"

"No. No one does." He says and grins again. I really dislike him when he grins. He sees the confusion in my face and leans forward, just an inch or two above me. "That little pathetic excuse for a bar owner?" He grins. "My men took care of that. And his goons. And - " there is a stupid, exaggerated theatrically in his pauses that I find really annoying. "Some of the poor unfortunates who frequented his establishment at that time."

"You killed them all?" I find it incredible. Even in the Hub where Regulator justice is rarely questioned you can't just do whatever you want.

"There was a little industrial accident with some cables and a few unfortunately contraband substances, it would appear."

He says. He's really full of himself with pride. "All that's left is a charred husk of a place and carbonized bodies inside."

"You bastard!" It's an unnecessary loss of life. I know what's coming next.

"And Snug, of course. How unfortunate that he dealt in exotic weaponry. There's nothing but small piles of red dust swirling in his shop."

"How convenient."

"The Hub is not a very friendly place," he grins again and I notice now just how cold that grin really is.

"Anyway, enough talk. We have plans for you Reaper." He motions to the Lab Tech and the man turns away to do something in his console. I hear the whirring of robotic arms just behind my head and I force myself to not react. I will not give the Jackal the pleasure of seeing me struggle. "Prep him. Execute," he tells the man and with a sharp click of his heels he turns around and walks away.

The robotic arms whirr above me.

"Don't worry," the Lab Tech says surprisingly soothingly to me. "You won't feel a thing." There's a jab in my arm where he's injected me with something and everything goes a little fuzzy.

I don't exactly pass out but nothing is quite lucid either. I come to and there are dozens of needles stuck in me. My neck, arms, torso. I am naked and strapped down. There's the smell of blood in the air or maybe that's only inside my head. I don't really know any more. I feel nothing. My body is not my own.

"Gene splicing at this level is an art," the Lab Tech talks as he works. His hands fly over buttons on consoles like a consummate pianist. "Tessa was a true artist in this. She's been sequencing genomes and splicing them, switching on and off arcane genes for years. She was a true master. But even a master needs a good canvas to work with. Something amazing. We've been looking for the right material for so long now. Sometimes, when we got lucky in the past, the technique was not quite so refined. At other times we overlooked something minor. A tiny expressive gene that turned out to be major. We learnt the hard way, the hardest way possible actually. You're lucky."

"Lucky?" I can barely contain my mirth and, talking as it turns out, is the only thing I can do.

"I know you don't think so but we looked at the samples Tessa send us on you. You're perfect. Even more perfect than that little girl and she got away. But we'll get her back."

"Ellie?"

"I don't know her name. The Captain will find her. He finds everybody. That's his special skill."

"Right."

"But back to you my friend. You will find that you will fade in and out. Don't worry. That's normal. No pain. But as the genes take effect there will be changes. You will notice yourself fading. There is some exotic material there," he says with real pride in his voice, "once it takes effect you will slowly disappear."

"What do you hope to accomplish?" I ask, "If I am as rare as you say then all you have is just one. One Chimera."

"Oh, you don't understand. We will have the recipe. We can clone you forever. An unbeatable army we can control."

"You will never control me," I say.

"Carry on believing that," he smirks. Then, as he turns a switch, "see you on the other side Reaper."

I am fighting against the restraints that hold me down. Muscles ripple, sinews heave, tendons tense. I almost hear bones cracking and teeth chipping as I pit everything I am, everything I have against the fate reserved for me.

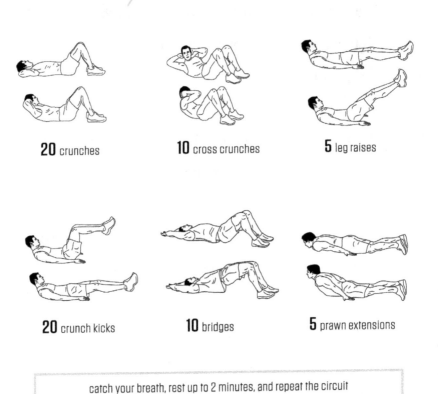

20 crunches   **10** cross crunches   **5** leg raises

20 crunch kicks   **10** bridges   **5** prawn extensions

catch your breath, rest up to 2 minutes, and repeat the circuit
3 times in total

Pain. Pain is a constant. I blank it out. Fear. I am really afraid. Inside my head there is a heavy, frightening growl. Something huge and fast with teeth and claws is coming my way and it really wants me dead. I hide. Darkness shields me from it.

I find myself running in darkness. Trying to outpace a terror that doesn't tire and doesn't stop.

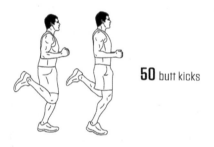

50 butt kicks

I run and run until my legs cannot carry me. I fall and fade. Cry and feel pain.

I am on Eden. My paradise retirement place. I try to make amends for those I killed. Give something back to those I come in contact with. I find myself endlessly lifting heavy boulders, taking them away from the beach.

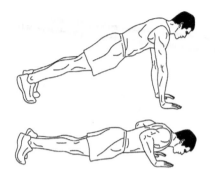

10 push-ups

catch your breath

10 push-ups

catch your breath

10 push-ups

It's hard work and the sun is ferociously hot and I am thirsty but I can't stop. I bring boulder after boulder but when I look back the boulders have somehow returned to the beach and I have to bring them all back again. I cry out. Feel Pain. Then fade.

In the final test I am climbing. A sheer rock face. No rope. Only hands and feet. I have to use my core. Abs to pull myself up again and again.

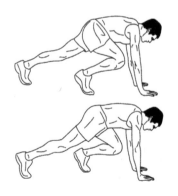

20 climbers

catch your breath

20 climbers

catch your breath

20 climbers

Look for handholds and footholds where they barely exist. I don't look down. I am really high. I cling desperately to the rock face, back muscles aching. Abs burning. My hands and feet are numb. Cut and bleeding. I hold on. Abs on fire. The tension is incredible. Something begins to give. A muscle in my lower back locks. My glutes cry out.

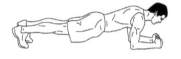

2 Minutes elbow plank hold

I can no longer hold on. I begin to fall. Slow motion. I fade.

Fade. Fade.

"Well? We got it?" I understand the words. I don't know where I am. I blink to clear my eyes. It's some sort of long cargo hold. Metal bulkheads everywhere. Tiny, intercom voices filtering to me. I realize no one is talking to me. I can overhear things.

"Yes sir. We finally have it."

"Show me."

"Look up please." Says an incredibly loud and very polite voice. I recognize it as the Lab Tech but it is so very loud now. I look up and see above me a series of metal rings. They are embedded in the ceiling overhead. "Jump up and grab them please," I don't think about it. I just do it.

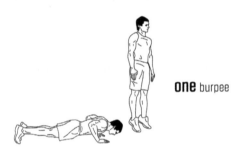

one burpee

The leap is easily forty feet. It almost feels like flying. One moment I am standing at ground level, looking up. The next I am holding onto the rings. Feet dangling. "Let go please," the voice says. It is coming from a loudspeaker. My hands open.

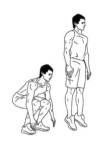

one jump squat

I drop down, land smoothly with barely a thud.

There are more commands. I bend metal and crack
bulletproof glass. I run across the cargo hold and cartwheel
in midair. I perform on command. Throw heavy things about
that I have no right to even lift. Something metal and heavy
comes at me powered by a robotic arm and I seize it in mid-
flight. Stop it dead with lightning-fast reflexes and I bend
it in half. The tests go on and on and on. The commanding
voice mesmerizing.

"Impressive," from the Jackal this time. How do I know all
this? "We have total control?"

"Yes sir. The sequencing led us to a restructured reward

system. That makes motivation subject to obedience which triggers hypothalamic responses. It's a little more complex but basically it takes pleasure in obeying us. We imprint voice modulation so only specific people can command it."

"Right. Right. All this will hold through cloning?"

"We don't know yet sir. Theoretically yes. But until we clone several, look for any unexpected deficiencies or micro-mutations that change things..."

"Right. Right. Do it. Do it tonight. We need to know asap."

"Sir."

I stand. Dumbly waiting for some command to obey.

Darkness. The things I fear. Death is not one of them. I fear vanishing. Disappearing without a trace, leaving nothing behind. Dissolution means meaninglessness. It's like life means nothing. I fear madness. Actions without logic. I fear darkness. The kind of darkness that steals me from my head.

I don't know how to explain what happens next. Some of the articulation I had has left me. It is hard to put thoughts into words. But some other things are easier. I can almost see genes inside me. Not see them. I am aware of them. It's like I can adapt to order. My orders. Adapt to overcome. I can see, for instance, how epigenetic changes affect imprinting, create neural circuits that bypass higher executive functions, robbing me of free will. Choice. And I can change that. If I wish.

I wish.

Change.

What happens next.

I am immune to cold and pain. Energy weapons can kill me but they have to hit me full on. I am fast. Really fast. And strong. Very strong. Space can't kill me. I don't even need oxygen to survive. I cannot explain this because I breathe. But out in space I don't have to. I can feel the radiation. Warm against my skin. And I am big. Larger than humans are.

What happened.

Metal is torn up. I rage.

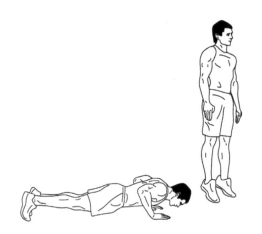

10 burpees

catch your breath

10 burpees

catch your breath

10 burpees

catch your breath

10 burpees

catch your breath

10 burpees

Claxons. I find flesh is soft. Pulpy. Even bones. They smash easily against metal bulkheads.

What happened. Flashing lights. Air escaping as the ship depressurizes. Bulkheads smashed. Cold. Darkness. Fear. Chaos.

Destruction. Death.

Everyone dies. An unmarked ship in an unauthorized orbit. I know the planet below is the Hub. I like the Hub. I have met people there I did not want to kill. The ship is full of blood. Bodies. On several walls written in human blood I have left them all a message. A legend:

RED REAPER.

Epilogue

Every system is dependent upon its limitations. They control what happens to that system and they govern the economic behavior of the system's participants.

Xelium was a defining element that factored in every decision. But the Ellie Transfer Drive changed all of that. Capable of manufacturing Xelium from cheap raw materials fed directly into the drive it untethered everyone from the Xelium cartels and led to the collapse of the Corporations.

History tells us that it was Dr. J. T. Ri who developed it but it was his daughter who managed to get the secret he'd discovered out safely and then into the hands of those who could spread it across the galaxy. The drive was named after her to honor her struggle.

It was her two companions, a hacker and a Regulator who got her hooked up to the network. The secret, encoded within her own DNA all along, was broadcast across all frequencies in the galaxy.

Ships fly today anywhere they want. There are no mining planets because mining is a thing of the past. There are no energy corporations because energy is plentiful. Humans, of course, being human constantly find new ways to create bottlenecks in the civilizations they create. But most of those are by choice and those who live by the parameters these bottlenecks impose have long made their peace with limiting principles and scarcity models.

The rest of humanity is finally free. As ships spread far
and wide across the known universe tales have come
back through the grapevine. Ships in trouble, helped.
Occasional acts of piracy thwarted. The tales speak of an
anthropomorphic entity swimming in from space. Helping
when help is needed. Stopping acts of aggression by a sheer
exhibition of immense power. Then vanishing again.

Nonsense of course. In all the known universe mankind has
never encountered alien lifeforms of any kind. Still. The
rumors persist. Grown men swear at what they have seen in
bars all over the planets and then, they reach for a drink.

Captains are a superstitious lot. They all have emergency
beacons set to emit on all frequencies a pre-arranged signal
based on Earth's old Morse:

three dots
one dot
two dots a dash and a dot

For those whose Morse is a little rusty the signal spells out:
SEF.

Thank you!

Thank you for purchasing **Carbon & Dust: 30-Day RPG Fitness**, DAREBEE project print edition. DAREBEE is a non-profit global fitness resource dedicated to making fitness accessible for everyone, no matter their circumstances. The project is supported exclusively via user donations and paperback royalties.

After printing costs and store fees every book developed by the DAREBEE project makes $1 and it goes directly into our project maintenance and development fund.

Each sale helps us keep the DAREBEE resource growing, maintain it and keep it up. Thank you for making a difference in its future!

Other books in this series include:

100 No-Equipment Workouts Vol 1.
100 No-Equipment Workouts Vol 2.
100 No-Equipment Workouts Vol 3.
100 HIIT Workouts
100 Office Workouts
Pocket Workouts: 100 no-equipment workouts
ABS 100 Workouts: Visual Easy-To-Follow ABS Exercise Routines for All Fitness Levels

Glossary

Ancient Archives: The repositories of the Histories. Everything that has been compiled, scavenged and saved of the human universe. The Archives are incomplete and those who study them have to have tutors and exercise strong inference to understand them.

Andromeda 6: One of the thriving service industry planets. Mostly finance and commerce theory but it also fields a couple of War Academies that have managed to make a name for themselves.

Carbide Trade-Off: Named after the defunct Terran Corp, Union Carbide, the Carbide trade-off is called this way because of the sensitive nature of its sequencing. In some exotic conditions the cycle can become unstable and the drive can implode. Fortunately this happens in extremely rare circumstances.

Chimeras: A chimera is essentially a single organism that's made up of cells from two or more "individuals"—that is, it contains two sets of DNA, with the code to make two separate organisms.

Cloaking field: A highly technical field force device that uses quantum effect to manipulate light so that the field acts like a highly sensitive photoconductor. Basically it projects what is on one side of it to the other and it does so in every direction. Its main characteristic is that it renders the subject inside the field virtually invisible.

Corporate High Language: Based upon ancient English this highly mutated but effective form of communication has been adopted as the HQ language of every Corporation in the known universe because it is easy to learn and adaptable enough to contain ambiguity even in its strictest expression. Something that comes in handy during business negotiations and trade deals.

Corporate Planetary Explorer: All Corporations have agreed that Explorers fly under a neutral flag. Their uniform then marks them to be respected and never be subjected to hostilities.

Corporation Wars: The Corporation Wars sprung out of Old Earth animosities. Corporations, wealthy beyond imagining, found themselves acquiring mercenaries and launching armed skirmishes with rivals in a bid to weaken their grip on specific markets. It soon escalated into a massive intergalactic conflict that bankrupted quite a few of them.

Digiplaque: Old tech. Hard to fake. Bonded metal with built-in memory and data storage capabilities. Primarily used as letters of credit or expensive, non-transferable, off-world tickets.

Electro-bonds: Nanosynth binders that hold an electric charge. The charge changes the load parameters of the material's matrix, making them virtually unbreakable. They are used by both law enforcement and military outfits to immobilize captive personnel.

Exoskeleton: Synth suits that end in gloves and boots. They are fluid metal that hardens on impact making them deadly in combat. They are powered by body heat and an internal battery pack. Expensive but useful, though they are not sufficiently hardened to withstand modern army weaponry. This has rendered them mostly obsolete.

Ghost Ship: Occasionally, in space, a ship is found. Empty, drifting. The crew vanished without explanation. Legends have grown around these finds. Space wraiths and exotic energies. Space pirates and space madness. No one knows for sure because no one talks about them. So the rumors persist. The legends grow through whispers.

GT planets: Mining designation. GT planets have a rich ore deposit. They are usually Xelium-rich. This makes them exploitable. Corporations always invest the bare minimum required for the maximum return.

GT-701: A hub mining planet. With a largely exhausted Xelium mining core it has found a new life as a transport hub for all sorts of cargo that skirts the legality of Corporation Law.

GX Dialect: Galactic Exchange is a standard language used for Corporate communication, trade deals and negotiations. It is based on old English-sans any hint of romanticism. Its high level of mabiguity makes it particularly well-suited for Corporate communication.

Healing Pod: Advanced medical tech that uses special magnetic fields and novel genetic material to speed up the body's healing process. There are rumors of side-effects that come as the result of frequent use which limits their effectiveness in one's lifespan, but for those odd occasions when rapid healing is required they are unparalleled.

Heat charge: Synthetic molecular hyper-activator. Every explosive device known to man employs the same principle of rapid energy expansion that outstrips its steady-state form. Heat charges employ a unique nanomolecule configuration that packs solid state material in a complex matrix of incredible density. The molecular bonds require an initial charge to activate them that is provided by traditional ammonium nitrate explosives. Once triggered, depending on the specific configuration they can achieve a detonation velocity that outstrips any other explosive agent.

Holomap: Old tech but effective. 3D-projections of topologies. Useful when offline with no access to online maps.
Hub-1: as the name implies a hub transportation planet by locale that's been configured to handle heavy interspace traffic. This is trickier than you might think. There are specific requirements for facilities designed to dock, repair (if necessary) and make space-ready again ships that have come in from deep space.

Hypermod: A heavily modified human. When it comes to human modification you usually get two competing ideologies. The first is called Augs. They are naturally (or biochemically) augmented humans. The second is called Mods. They are mechanically modified via implants and biosurgery. Hypermods straddle two worlds and form a class of their own. Their bodies are receptacles of enhancements and augmentations of all types.

Nano-tech suit: An advanced type of spacesuit that forms a hermetically sealed, self-sustaining, protective barrier around its wearer.

Orion Massacre: One of the bloodiest massacres in Galactic History. An entire mining planet's colony wiped out alongside a Regulator detachment sent to protect them. Corporations strongly condemned the attack. Although officially it remained a mystery the suggestion is that it was the first appearance of the Red Reaper, the most notorious assassin in the human universe.

Oxygen Gangs: In poor worlds where terraforming has not yet been completed the amount of oxygen that is available is strictly rationed. This has created a criminal underclass where gangs intercept shipments of oxygen and sell them for profit.

Pulverizer: Starting life as a mining implement intended to smash rocks into dust the pulverizer was soon modified into a weapon which, officially, all Corporations have outlawed.

Red Reaper: The most wanted (and feared) assassin-for-hire in the galaxy. No one knows what he really looks like and some even say that he's a myth. A made-up persona created to conveniently pin on, crimes that have to remain unsolved. There is a massive reward out for his capture and an all-Colonies alert.

Regulators: The closest thing the galaxy has to a universal police force and army. On some colonies Regulators are nothing more than policemen. But they are also the legal army of all Corporations. They act as a military force against rebel forces and terrorists. Because all Corporations pull Regulators from the same general pool it makes it difficult for them to really go into war against each other. Regulators then, perversely, manage to keep intergalactic peace.

RIM Corp: In old Terra, RIM was a tech company associated with personal communication devices. It is now one of the galaxy's most feared corporations. Its name synonymous with might and, occasionally, practices that sail a little too close to the edge of legality for comfort.

Sanctuary: Even in space there is need for oases. A sanctuary is a retrofitted space platform that has been engineered to provide living quarters, refueling stations, dock repairs and so on. Sanctuaries are enterprises. They bridge deep space between the ever expanding GT mining planet network. They cost the corporations little and deliver a valuable service so their legal status is never questioned. They are treated, instead, as strictly neutral points in space.

The Lords of Mirth: Old cult religion that was exported from Orion to most of the known Galaxy. Its basic tenet is that the universe has a sense of humor and it exercises it at the expense of its human occupants. "Make all the plans you want" goes the popular adage, "The Lords of Mirth only laugh louder."

The Wired: A secretive and legendary order of Hypermods living in seclusion and only occasionally venturing into human space. They almost never get involved in human affairs. Not much is known about them.

Tolarian: Ancient tongue whose last foothold was on Orion. It is distantly related to the click language of old Terra, known as Khoisan.

Type-C cargo ship: A massive cargo hold divided into compartments with two massive engines stuck on it. Type-C cargo ships are the container ships of space. Very uncomfortable for space travel but very profitable for the transportation of goods. The one glaring problem they have is that they are designed to be repaired while in dock. They are designed to take damage but anything that really damages them in space is very likely to cause them to end.

War Academy: As the name suggests, educational establishments specifically created to train and educate Regulators.

Wormhole fever: There is a contention amongst cognitive scholars whether there is such a thing as wormhole fever. Ships' captains who have seen it first hand in their crew however do not doubt that the mini-psychotic episodes they see are the strain of a human brain jumping too many times into the heart of spacetime.

Xelium: The ultimate currency of the galaxy. Xelium is mined, for fuel, everywhere and without it the galaxy and all its creations would grind to a halt. Its presence underpins all existing socio-economic and political power structures.

9 781844 810185